PRAISE FOR
PAIN-FREE WITH MAGNET THERAPY

"With easy-reading intelligence, Lara Owen guides us between narrow-minded skepticism and overblown hype to reveal what every consumer and professional needs to know about magnet therapy. Her balanced exposition of magnet therapy is most timely. The book achieves magnificently its goal of providing the consumer and professional alike with the information necessary to make wise decisions. At last, an unbiased and in-depth book on magnet therapy that will become indispensable to both consumers and professionals."

—Michael Waterhouse, M.A., L.Ac.,
clinical instructor, U.C.L.A.,
Department of Pediatrics

"A valuable contribution to the literature on magnet therapy. Written from an acupuncturist's perspective, it will be particularly interesting to health-care professionals working in the field of energy medicine."

—Agatha P. Colbert, M.D.

"Magnets are helping a great number of people, and Lara Owen has written an excellent book that provides scientific insight into how effective magnets really are."

—Daniel Man, M.D

Pain-Free with Magnet Therapy

Pain-Free with Magnet Therapy

Discover How Magnets Can Help Relieve Arthritis, Sports Injuries, Fibromyalgia, and Chronic Pain

LARA OWEN

PRIMA HEALTH
A Division of Prima Publishing
3000 Lava Ridge Court • Roseville, California 95661
(800) 632-8676, ext. 4444 • www.primahealth.com

PRIMA HEALTH and colophon are trademarks of Prima Communications Inc., registered with the United States Patent and Trademark Office.

Library of Congress Cataloging-in-Publication Data
Owen, Lara.
    Pain-free with magnet therapy : discover how magnets can help relieve arthritis, sports injuries, fibromyalgia, and chronic pain / Lara Owen.
    p. cm.
Includes bibliographical references and index.
ISBN 0-7615-2086-4
1. Magnetotherapy. 2. Chronic pain. I. Title.

RM893.O944 2000
615.8′45—dc21   00-026820

00 01 02 03 HH 10 9 8 7 6 5 4 3 2
Printed in the United States of America

How to Order
Single copies may be ordered from Prima Publishing, 3000 Lava Ridge Court, Roseville, CA 95661; telephone (800) 632-8676, ext. 4444. Quantity discounts are also available. On your letterhead, include information con-cerning the intended use of the books and the number of books you wish to purchase.

Visit us online at www.primahealth.com

Contents

Part 3 Practical Applications

Part 4 Theories and Speculation

Foreword

"I predict we will see the day when all humans will be able to walk into something resembling a telephone booth, be scanned with complex electromagnetic fields, receive a diagnosis such as 'Several cells in your liver are sick,' and be instantly treated by an electromagnetic field specifically configured to cure those cells." This was said to me by an orthopedic surgeon, the late C. Andrew L. Bassett, in the early 1970s while we were collaborating together at Columbia University to develop pulsing electromagnetic fields for the treatment of difficult-to-heal bone fractures. Obviously the day that Andy Bassett predicted has not yet arrived and is still far in the future, but not as far as it was then. This book is testament to that.

The use of magnetic fields for therapeutic purposes has not been without controversy and skepticism. Many anecdotal reports of this or that specific field curing cancer, arthritis, baldness, or any of a host of other pathologies gave magnetic fields the reputation of snake oil. This reputation changed, however, when in the mid-1960s orthopedic researchers began wondering how bone could structurally adapt to mechanical stresses. Why was it that people who rode horses all day became bowlegged? Why did the forearm bones of a professional tennis player become thicker than those of the average person? The answer turned out to be that bone structure adaptively responds to mechanical stresses through an electromagnetic process.

This answer led to the reemergence of pulsing magnetic fields as a credible therapeutic modality in the 1970s, at least for bone fractures. Pulsing magnetic fields for the treatment of bone fractures are currently employed by orthopedic surgeons worldwide. The field of magnetic therapy has had its share of growing pains. "Show me the double-blind studies." "How does it work?" "It can only be a heating effect." These are some of the issues driving research in the field, even as this is being written. Fortunately, research in the biophysics and biology of magnetic fields has developed to the point that credibility is much less of an issue. In fact, specific venues have been created for the peer review of studies in magnetic field bioeffects. Several professional societies and specialized journals are now well-established. Static magnetic field therapy benefits from all of this.

Does this mean that we now know enough to state that simple static magnets are the answer to all your aches and pains? Not yet! There are still many, many unknowns, and Lara Owen has done a superb job of guiding you through the current facts and fictions of static magnet therapeutics. The word has gotten around that many people have reported that magnets have relieved their particular pain. This has opened a huge market, and there is money to be made selling magnets for all parts of the body. The economic stakes are high, and the marketeers are claiming that magnets heal everything. Fortunately for you and the professionals, the FDA, via the FTC, has stopped the more outrageous of the claims, particularly on the Web. But the FDA doesn't practice medicine and doesn't do the clinical trials necessary to establish the efficacy of magnetic treatment for a particular malady. The FDA expects those who make the claims, the vendors, to do this. But it is not only the FDA that needs to be satisfied. In general, clinicians are a bunch of skeptics and need to have double-blind or convincing case studies. The positive side of all of this skepticism and regulation means that proper clinical evaluations are being done on static magnet therapy. The available results are presented and analyzed in this book.

Among the most important questions you face in choosing a magnet or magnetic device are those related to dose: How much? How long? Although there are no complete answers yet, Lara takes you through what is known and unknown in sufficient detail for you to make an informed decision. The present state of knowledge certainly suggests that static magnets could help render you pain free. It certainly is worth a try, and if you do get relief, then my dream of a world in which electromagnetic fields play an important therapeutic role comes closer to reality.

Thank you Lara Owen for making the technical and biological complexities of magnet therapy realistically accessible to all who are searching for help.

—Arthur A. Pilla, Ph.D.

Department of Orthopedics
Mount Sinai School of Medicine, New York

Department of Biomedical Engineering
Columbia University, New York

Acknowledgments

Many people helped me in various ways with this book, and I am most grateful to everyone who took the time to answer my questions and share the experiences they've had with magnets. Special thanks are due to Arthur Pilla, who was enormously helpful, kindly answering my endless questions and giving me a great deal of assistance with scientific accuracy, as well as introducing me to other researchers in the field. Many thanks also to Keith Kirk, who patiently explained much of the science of magnets and magnetism to me. I also want to especially thank Diane Black, Steven Bratman, Agatha Colbert, Elizabeth DuBois, Holly Guzman, Richard Hammerschlag, Carlton Hazlewood, Daniel Man, James Moran, and Michael Waterhouse—all of whom went out of their way to send me information, give me research leads, and, in some cases, review parts of the manuscript.

Introduction

Everywhere one looks these days, there are therapeutic magnets—on sale in Kmart and Target, on the Shopping Channel, strapped to the wrists of golf pros, and featured on many Web sites. Magnet sales are booming. But is there really anything to them? Are magnets just another form of pseudomedical hype? This book will answer these questions and help you make informed decisions about whether using magnets might be a useful avenue for you to explore.

Fortunately for all of us, magnet therapy is a rapidly growing area of medical research, fueled by a growing public interest. More and more people are choosing to use magnets to relieve their chronic aches and pains. They find that magnets give them pain relief without the side effects of analgesic drugs.

There is also evidence that magnets may have other exciting therapeutic possibilities. Magnet therapy is being used as a treatment for the symptoms of several diseases, including fibromyalgia and diabetes. Magnets are increasingly used for sports injuries and for treating injured horses and arthritic dogs. Magnets are also used in special mattress pads that are said to enhance sleep as well as ease aches and pains—although, of course, when you don't have pain, you sleep better anyway. When you sleep well, your overall health tends to improve, which is why proponents of magnetic sleep therapy say that it boosts the immune system.

The most extreme enthusiasists claim that magnets act as a universal panacea that can totally transform your health and well-being. This hyperbole may seem new to us, but it's not without precedent. Throughout history, there have been times when there was as much conjecture and excitement about magnets as there is today, but without any hard evidence to back up the enthusiasm.

Today, we are in a different situation. With modern scientific techniques, we can assess how effective magnet therapy actually is. We can check for side effects. We can test all the speculative theories in order to separate fantasy from reality. We can have the best of both worlds: by combining ancient folklore with modern scientific method, we have the chance to use a relatively inexpensive healing tool with effectiveness and accuracy.

Several well-designed research studies on magnets have recently been completed, and many more are underway. We are finally beginning to have some reliable, factual evidence about how magnets can help us. In this book, we're going to look at all the claims for magnet therapy in the light of recent scientific evidence. This will give you the most factually grounded understanding of magnet therapy available at the present time.

Part 1

Introduction to Magnet Therapy

1

What Is Magnet Therapy?

In brief, magnet therapy is the practice of using magnets of various strengths on different body parts in order to produce a healing effect in a variety of conditions. Magnet therapy has been around for thousands of years in one form or another and is currently enjoying a big revival.

This book focuses on the kind of magnets that you place next to your body. These magnets are called permanent, or static, magnets. These are the magnets that are for sale in stores, on television shopping channels, on the Internet, and through multilevel marketing companies. Many people use these magnets without necessarily seeking the guidance of medical experts.

Another area of magnetic therapy currently receiving considerable attention by researchers is the use of pulsing electromagnetic fields, which at the moment require sophisticated machines and have to be applied by a physician. (See chapter 9 for a more complete discussion of this type of magnet therapy.)

Therapeutic magnets of the permanent variety can be small and strong in intensity, for dealing with acute injury or severe localized pain, or they can be contained in a large pad that covers an area of the body, such as the lower back. Mattress pads filled with hundreds of tiny magnets are also becoming popular.

Magnets are gradually becoming accepted in the scientific community. There are an increasing number of scientific studies supporting the use of magnets (see part 2), and there are an abundance of theories about how and why magnets work (see chapter 15). Before delving further into the scientific detail of magnet therapy, let's take a look at some magnet stories and background information on magnets and magnet therapy from the present as well as the distant past.

STORIES OF MAGNET THERAPY

I'll start with the story of how I came to write this book. In the spring of 1999, Prima Publishing approached me about writing a book on magnet therapy. Prima came to me for two reasons. First, because I had done some previous work with them and had written other health-related books; and second, because I have a background in acupuncture. (As you will see later in this book, there is a longstanding relationship between the energy-based practice of acupuncture and the therapeutic use of magnets.) However, I had never used magnets myself and knew little about how they worked or even if they worked. I had a dim recollection of high school physics experiments, but other than that I knew nothing about the science of magnets. A little daunted by my own ignorance on the subject, I nonetheless accepted the assignment, as I suspected that the subject would intrigue me.

I also knew that I could be more objective than someone more invested in magnets, either professionally or financially. I felt that objectivity was important in a field that appeared to be rife with conjecture and hype. This feeling turned out to be very true, and I spent several months wading through misleading Web sites and exaggerated claims in other books.

Another factor that drew me toward this subject was the larger picture of how healing methods reflect and inform human culture. New forms of healing (even if they are apparently based on something old) are of great interest to me, both in terms of what they can realistically offer us and as an insight into the future development and the hopes and dreams of humankind. I knew that if magnets really did work, and if scientists were beginning to understand how, then this knowledge might be a key to unlocking some of the mystery surrounding other remedies that are not explained by the current consensus about the minds and bodies of human beings, such as acupuncture and homeopathy.

If you have used therapeutic magnets yourself, you already know more about using magnets than I did when I started doing research for this book. If you are still intrigued by magnets after using them, the odds are that they helped you and you want to find out more about them. This book will help to fill out your knowledge and answer some of your questions. If you have never used magnets before and are thinking about trying them, the book will tell you what you need to know in order to make an informed decision.

After I took the assignment and started telling my friends about it, I was amazed to discover how many of them were already using magnets. One friend was using a pair of magnetic foot insoles to help with the side effects of sitting in front of a computer all day; another had used a magnet to cure cellulite on her thigh; another had been sleeping on a huge magnet under his mattress for five years and was sure it gave him more energy. (All these stories are told in more detail in later chapters.) Another friend, this time someone who was completely against using Western medicine, tried to cure herself of pneumonia by using magnets. Her attempt was not successful, and she became very ill. This is a cautionary tale for those of us who might be tempted to ignore a serious symptom and use a magnet instead of going to the doctor. Magnet therapy should never be used as a substitute for proper medical care.

As I listened to all these tales, I realized that something potentially very important was happening. If magnets really were effective in relieving pain and in somehow stimulating the flow of energy in the body, then magnets could have a substantial impact on how we deal with inflammation, pain, and a host of other conditions. But I had many questions. Were magnets safe? Did people know how to use magnets properly? Did anyone have a clue about how magnets worked? What research was being done? Was there any hard evidence at all that magnets were anything more than a pseudoscientific placebo?

To answer these questions, and many more, in the summer of 1999 I began doing intensive research. I turned first to the modern researcher's favorite—and sometimes unreliable—tool: the Internet. There I found a wealth of Web sites on magnets—some that seemed ethical and informative, and some that made me nervous, that made all kinds of wild claims substantiated with data of dubious origin. This research gave me a taste of the amount of marketing energy going into selling magnets, and it also indicated that for all these mail-order businesses to be springing up, there must be a substantial demand for magnet therapy. It was also clear that the claims made by some Web sites were going to entice some people to part with their money more out of hope and desperation than out of any grounded information about magnets. Later that summer the Federal Trade Commission cracked down on these sites and ordered changes in many of them. As a result, by late 1999, the tenor of most of the Web sites was more measured than it had been earlier in the year.

One day, in a moment of boredom, I turned on the television. As I idly channel-surfed, I came across an hour-long special about magnets on the QVC shopping channel. People were calling in from all over the country, claiming that wearing magnets had helped everything from gout to multiple sclerosis. One woman said she was walking again after having been confined to a wheelchair. All my suspicions were aroused. I wondered if these people were real or if the whole thing was a big set-up. At that point, I thought that the magnet business seemed exactly that—a big business, which, like so many health-related scams before it, was feeding off the fears and needs of the public. There's always a tacky atmosphere invoked when money, salesmanship, and the hope of an easy cure-all occur in the same moment, or in this case, the same infomercial. I began to feel disheartened and realized it was time to change tack and talk to people who were actually using magnets.

I wanted to talk to laypeople, doctors, acupuncturists, veterinarians, and whoever else was using magnets as part of a healing modality. I also wanted to interview scientists who were doing research into the physics of magnets and how it relates to the body. During the following six months, I met many people and conducted scores of phone interviews.

Research is like following a trail. One person leads you to another, until you have colored in a whole picture with the pieces that make up its totality. With a field like magnet therapy, however, it is impossible to get to totality, because the landscape is constantly evolving. At some point you have to stop and write the whole thing up. But along the way, a certain logic of discovery comes into play, and the characters and themes gradually emerge until the picture comes into focus. On this particular research journey, it was the laypeople who had experienced beneficial effects who turned up first and told me their stories, so that is where I will begin.

I was sitting at my desk, wondering how to go about meeting people who had used magnets, when a friend arrived at my door. She had come to tell me that she had just been at a party and had met a woman who seemed to know a great deal about magnets. I called the woman from the party, and this is her story. (Throughout the book, the names of laypeople who use magnets have been changed to protect their privacy.)

Annie

Annie is in her late thirties and lives in a small California town with her husband and daughter. She suffered from constant back pain for nine years. She had been a nurse, and she thinks that lifting patients may have caused her back condition. Annie's orthopedic doctor and chiropractor felt they had done as much as they could, and she was beginning to despair. She woke every morning in pain. Her only alternative to chronic, debilitating pain appeared to be surgery. As a registered nurse, she had seen enough of back surgery to have little faith in it as a cure for her condition.

Annie also felt tired much of the time and had been suffering from chronic fatigue syndrome for the past two years. One day, while at her three-year-old daughter's toddler group, she complained volubly to a friend about having no energy. A woman overheard her and suggested that she try sleeping on a magnetic mattress pad. Annie was skeptical but decided that she might as well try it, as she was fed up with feeling so tired all the time. She never expected it to help her back.

> I spent the night sleeping on the pad. In the morning, I got out of bed and, after a couple of seconds, realized that for the first time in nine years I had no back pain. I looked back at the bed and said, "Oh my gosh, my back doesn't hurt, what is this?"

> I called the woman and said, "Can magnets help back pain?" And she said yes. I couldn't believe it.

For Annie, the immediate relief from back pain seemed little short of miraculous. After that first night, she started using magnets every day to help her back condition. For three months nonstop, she wore a large magnet taped to her back during her waking hours. After that she used the magnet whenever she felt it was necessary. She bought the magnetic mattress pad and slept on it every night. She also wore magnetic insoles in her shoes. Now, a year later, she has very little discomfort in her back.

Annie's life is very active. She runs her own business while raising her daughter. These days she rarely needs to use the large back magnet during the day. She only uses it if some exertion has aggravated her back condition or if she knows she is going to be exerting herself. She continues to use the insoles and sleeps on the magnetic mattress pad every night.

> I used to hurt ninety-nine percent of the time, and now I hurt one percent of the time. I use the back magnet if I have to lift things or if I ride horses, which I had to give up for many years. . . . It took a year for me to go from ninety-nine percent pain to one percent, which I think is fast. This is a real alternative to taking pain medication.

Annie considers that magnet therapy has changed her life. She feels that magnets not only helped her back pain but also ultimately healed it. Her chronic fatigue syndrome also improved during her first year of using magnets. Annie believes that the magnets actually give her more energy by stimulating her electromagnetic field. However, her improved energy could simply be due to the fact that she is moving around more now that she is free of pain. No study has yet measured something as difficult to determine as energy level. However, the belief that magnets improve vitality is not an uncommon testimony from magnet users.

The day after meeting Annie, I had to call another publishing company to discuss a book of mine that had come out the previous year. "What are you working on now?" asked the publicist. "I'm doing a book on magnets," I said. "Oh!" she exclaimed, "Magnets just changed my life!" So there was my next story.

Sarah

Sarah is in her early thirties and works for a publishing company. She was involved in a major car accident that left her with damage to her shoulder, ribs, and upper back. The pain was excruciating, and pain relievers made her nauseous, dizzy, and unable to work. Sarah became concerned that she was going to lose her job as a result of the pain from her injuries.

As a last resort her doctor, having just read a recent study on the use of magnets, suggested that she try them. Sarah went to a local acupuncturist who used magnets and had several sessions, during which he would leave the magnets on acupuncture points related to the sites of her injuries. She did not like the idea of acupuncture needles, and the acupuncturist said that was no problem; he would use magnets instead. The acupuncturist used special high-powered gold magnets that were left on the acupuncture points for about 30 minutes. Then he removed the magnets and taped much lower intensity magnets to the same acupuncture points. These smaller magnets were left in place for a week, until Sarah returned for her next session.

Within days Sarah experienced much less pain. She was able to return to work because the magnets had no side effects. Without the excruciating pain or the effects of the painkillers, her ability to concentrate returned. Her injuries continued to heal, and six months later she was free of pain.

As I found out over the next few months, these stories were fairly typical of the success stories that abound concerning magnets. Annie's pain had been chronic, meaning she had endured the pain for a long time, and it had looked like it would never go away. Sarah had pain from an acute injury, meaning the odds were that in time her body would heal, but to what extent and how long it would take were debatable.

In time, I would hear of even more dramatic stories than these, some of which were hard to believe, not that I doubted the sincerity of any of the tellers. A good example of such tales is Bob's story. Bob donated a kidney to his brother. After the transplant, Bob was told to expect a lot of difficulty and considerable discomfort. He was expected to take seven to ten days to recover before being able to leave the hospital. He began using magnets immediately after the surgery, having his sister-in-law massage his legs with magnets.

"I snapped right out of the anesthesia," Bob said. He also put a large flexible magnetized pad on his lower back; as a result, he needed no pain medication. Bob was able to leave the hospital after two days.

When you hear a dramatic story like Bob's, it's important to bear in mind that belief in the therapy itself can play a large part in the healing process. Bob's speedy recovery certainly could have happened because he believed it would happen. The magnets may have acted as a placebo that stimulated his ability to recover quickly from major surgery.

Then there was Jim, whose story I heard from his wife, Emily. Jim was in his sixties and had a long history of serious ill health. He had the kind of case history that makes you want to weep for all the suffering it contains. He had had diabetes for the past 3 years, had developed neuropathy, and had to have a toe removed. He had had arthritis for 33 years, high blood pressure for 24 years, and back problems for 15 years. In the previous 2 years, Jim had become completely bedridden, with bedsores, boils, and an open wound that would not heal.

Jim began using magnets at the insistence of his exhausted wife. He did not feel positive about using the magnets, had no belief that they would work, and only used them because his wife made him. Even so, Emily noticed a big difference in his personality the very next day. For some years he had been prone to negativity and self-pity. After helping him use the magnets, Emily said, "All of a sudden I saw the man I had married."

On the third day the bedsores improved, and after a couple of months they were gone completely. By the third month, the couple reported that Jim's right-sided paralysis had improved, as had his temper, his bowel movements, the strength in his arms, and the ability to feel sensation instead of numbness in his legs. Even his large moles disappeared, and his sagging cellulite-ridden skin cleared up. In addition, his weight dropped considerably.

Emily seemed utterly credible to me, although I must confess the story left me reeling. I couldn't believe all this came about from magnets. As I was to find out, and as I recount in more detail later in this book, many of Jim's complaints seem to be amenable to magnet therapy. One study has shown that magnets improve pain and numbness from diabetic neuropathy, several have shown that magnets help to heal wounds and sores, and others have shown that magnets can alleviate chronic pain. The effects on Jim's mood and general well-being could have occurred as a corollary to these other benefits. No studies have been done on the use of static magnets to relieve depression, although pulsing electromagnetic fields are successfully being used for this condition. One researcher, Dr. Agatha Colbert, is currently designing a study using static magnets for depression.

As a rule, the results of using magnets are more ordinary than Jim's story. I heard many more utterly believable stories of people with annoying aches and pains and swollen joints that became more manageable when they strapped a magnet onto their wrist or elbow or wherever they had a problem. As I met all these people and heard what magnets had done for them, I had to accept that something of a significant healing dimension was taking place, and I became increasingly interested in trying to understand what that was.

While investigating what was currently happening in magnet therapy, I was also digging around to find out what magnets had been used for historically, which is what chapter 2 is all about. My quest was to find out how we came to use magnets in the first place and whether there is any historical basis for the healing effects of magnets.

2

A History of
Magnet Therapy

"The stone has a soul since it moves iron."

Aristotle, 600 B.C.E., referring to
magnetite, naturally occurring magnetic
rock commonly found in Greece.

The therapy that helped Annie, Sarah, Bob, and Jim has been known about for thousands of years and is one of the oldest healing methods known to humankind. In one form or another, magnets have been used in many cultures for their therapeutic properties. However, the extent to which magnets were used to heal in the distant past is not known and may have been exaggerated in some of the recent literature on magnets.[1]

Ancient peoples had access to magnets in two ways. First, they used magnets that occur naturally. These magnets are found in the form of lodestones, which are a type of iron ore called magnetite. It is probable that ancient peoples used lodestones for healing purposes. We do have documentation that the Chinese were using magnetic stones in healing at least 2,000 years ago. Lodestone also occurs in powdered form, which, according to old Chinese texts, was also used in healing. The Thousand Ducat Prescriptions (A.D. 652) includes the recommendation, "Put the powder of magnet on the injury for painkiller and to stop bleeding."

Second, it is possible to magnetize certain metals by heating them and putting them next to a piece of magnetic rock. Even with the most rudimentary of forges, people long ago could make their own magnets. They did this by heating a piece of iron until the atoms became fluid and then by sticking the iron next to a chunk of lodestone. The iron would pick up the cellular structure of the magnetized rock and become a magnet itself.

The word *magnet* comes to us via Latin from the ancient Greek word *magnes,* which was a shortened form of *ho Magnes lithos* ("the Magnesian stone"). *Ho Magnes lithos* has two possible sources. Lucretius wrote in the first century B.C.E. that the term was derived from Magnesia, a mineral-rich region of Greece, where presumably there were lodestone deposits. Pliny the Elder said that *ho Magnes lithos* was derived from the name of the shepherd, Magnes, "the nails of whose shoes and the tip of whose staff stuck fast in a magnetic field while he pastured his flocks." (No pun intended, one imagines.)

Some books state that a 100,000-year-old iron ore mine found in Africa is proof that magnets have been used for healing since the dawn of time. However, this mine contained red iron ore, which is not the same as magnetite and is not naturally magnetic. Also, because it is oxidized (ochre is ferrous hydroxide), it cannot be magnetized by simply applying heat and aligning it with another magnetic rock. Although the ancient Africans were intentionally mining red iron ore, it was not for magnetic healing purposes. Instead, they used red iron ore ceremonially, because the red ochre produced by grinding it resembled the color of blood, the symbol for human life. It is fairly obvious that this use of iron has nothing to do with using magnetic rocks for healing.

ANCIENT CHINESE
REFERENCES TO MAGNET THERAPY

We know that the Chinese have used magnets for thousands of years, but we don't know for exactly how long, how often they used them, or with how much success. We can presume, because of the continued use of magnets over time, that they had some efficacy. However, we can also make a logical assumption that the Chinese found acupuncture needles and herbs to be more effective treatments, because far more attention is paid to these forms of medicine in Chinese medical literature. This assumption has to be tempered with the fact that until the nineteenth century doctors only had access to natural magnets (lodestone) or to magnets made in forges. These magnets were probably not as powerful as the therapeutic magnets we make and use today. We can't know what the ancient Chinese sages would have said about today's sophisticated magnet technology.

I asked several acupuncturists using magnets how they felt about the comparative effectiveness of magnets and needles. They all agreed that, in general, needles work faster but that magnets used correctly are just as effective for many conditions and, in some cases, are the preferred method of treatment. (For more on the specific methods of using magnets on acupuncture points, see chapter 12.)

The earliest complete text on Chinese medicine is the *Huang Di Nei Jing,* the Yellow Emperor's Classic of Internal Medicine (also sometimes called the Emperor's Internal Classic). This classical text, as we know it, dates from around 200 B.C.E. but claims to be a much earlier work, dating from at least 2000 B.C.E. Indeed, the book contains such detailed and complex information that it is not hard to believe that this system of medicine was already well established by 200 B.C.E. Some books

and Web sites on magnets claim that the earliest references to magnets are found in the Yellow Emperor's
Classic *(Nei Jing)*. However, as far as I have been able to
ascertain, there is no reference to magnets in the *Nei
Jing*. There are references in other old Chinese medical
texts, but only from ones that date from later times. The
first known reference to magnets in Chinese literature is
found in the *Shih-chi* (Historical Records), which was
the first history of China. The *Shih-chi*, written by Ssu-
ma Ch'ien (145–85 B.C.E.), contains a record of events
and personalities covering the previous two thousand
years. Ssu-ma Ch'ien was a Chinese astronomer, calen-
dar expert, and the first great historian of China. The
Shih-chi, which was completed in about 85 B.C.E. and
which took 18 years to produce[2], refers to the use of
magnet therapy in the treatment of fevers.[3]

Shen-Nung's *Materia Medica* (the Shen-Nung-
Pen-Ts'ao-Ching), written in the second century B.C.E.,
includes a clear description of the use of magnet therapy
for wind bi syndrome.[4] Wind bi is a kind of arthritis that
tends to move from joint to joint and is considered to
have originated in what the Chinese call the external
evil of wind. It is most similar to the condition called
rheumatoid arthritis in Western medicine.

In the sixth century A.D., the *Ming-Yi Bie-Lu*
(Special Records of Famous Physicians) stated, "Magnet
nourishes the Kidney, strengthens the bones, stops
thirst, cures boils and lymphadenopathy of tuberculosis,
calms down hysteria and infantile seizures."[5] In the
Ch'ien-Chin-Yoa-Fang (Thousand Golden Prescriptions),
Sun Ssu Miao (A.D. 581–682) reported using magnet therapy to treat bleeding and pain from cuts, stating that he
treated a wound by applying powdered magnet to it.[6] A
later Chinese text (from A.D. 1735[7]) recommended magnets for helping with problems of both hearing and sight.
"Nothing is better than magnet for sight of eyes. Put the
magnet in the pillow, eyesight will never decline."

Traditional Chinese medicine is based on the notion that an energy force called *chi* flows through the body along certain pathways, called meridians. Magnets, with their electrical energy of attraction and repulsion, easily fit in with this belief system. Like inserting metal needles and burning herbs on the acupuncture points (moxibustion), magnets are thought to stimulate the body's chi to move. In so doing, magnets promote healing where there has been stagnation. They may also act as a tonifying force on energy points that activate the body's own tendency toward self-healing and balance (homeostasis). This perspective on health and healing has remained a basic tenet of Chinese thought and practice for more than four thousand years. It is possibly the oldest consistent biophysical philosophy in human history. Later chapters in this book show how Chinese medicine and magnets are used together.

ANCIENT EGYPTIANS

The Ancient Egyptians reputedly wore magnets to increase their longevity and health. Some sources claim that they used magnets for headaches, gout, and dropsy. Cleopatra (69–30 B.C.E.) is said to have worn a polished lodestone on her third eye to maintain her beauty.[8] I have not been able to verify any of these anecdotes, so for now they should be taken as simply that—historical legend that may or may not be factual.

PARACELSUS

The chain of knowledge about magnets resurfaced in Europe in the work of Paracelsus, the famous and gifted medical practitioner whose ideas foreshadowed many of the later developments of Western medicine. Paracelsus

(1493–1541) was a remarkable figure—an itinerant and irascible scholar and physician who originated many new theories in his relatively short life and who had a profound effect on the future development of medicine.

Paracelsus developed the theory of similars, from which Hahnemann later created homeopathy. Paracelsus cured people of the plague by giving them pills containing minute amounts of their own excrement. He used mercury to treat syphilis long before the nature of infectious disease was understood. He decried the ways that wounds were conventionally treated, which was to pour boiling oil on to cauterize them or to allow a limb to become gangrenous and then amputate it. He advocated draining the wound, keeping it clean, and allowing it to heal by itself.

Perhaps most importantly, Paracelsus said that medicine should only be used if it has been shown to be effective, not just because it has been used traditionally. He was, in many respects, a father of modern medicine. However, he was also a mystic, and many of his theories became unpopular during the Age of Reason. These days, some of his ideas are once again becoming popular.

Paracelsus believed that all life was infused with an invisible fluid he called "mumia." He maintained that bodily fluids, such as including blood, sweat, and urine, carried this life essence and could be used in healing. He argued that healthy mumia could attract diseased mumia, rather like a magnet attracts iron. Along similar lines of thought, he experimented with using actual magnets on his patients and is reported to have cured women of hysterical disorders by placing the positive pole of a magnet at the head and the negative pole of another magnet "below", presumably over the uterus.[9]

The word "hysterical" comes from the Greek *hustera,* meaning "womb." Hysteria in women was a condition that engaged medical attention for several centuries and may have been caused as much by political reasons of suppression than by any physiological cause. Whatever the reason for the disorder, Paracelsus apparently was able to calm anxious women by using magnets in this way.

MESMER

Two centuries later, Franz Anton Mesmer expanded on the ideas of Paracelsus, and magnetism again became a source of interest and intrigue. Like Paracelsus, Mesmer used magnets on hysterical young women, a treatment for which he became famous and, later on, infamous.

Mesmer's theories about magnetism provide a fascinating glimpse into the early days of energy theory in the West. Some of his ideas share similarities with Chinese theories of *chi,* a system of thought to which he was most unlikely exposed, as it would be another two hundred years before Chinese medical texts would be translated into European languages.

Mesmer, the German doctor whose work gave us the term "mesmerism," was born in the small town of Iznang in 1734. He graduated in medicine from the University of Vienna, where he wrote a dissertation on the relationship between the planets and human disease, a subject that was not as bizarre as it might seem today. Mesmer lived in an era when scientific thinking, as we now know it, was just developing and when medicine was still infused with a sense of poetry and mysticism. In his dissertation, Mesmer suggested that the gravitational attraction of the planets influenced an invisible fluid found in all living things, including the human body. He later refined this theory into the concept he called animal magnetism.

Mesmer's breakthrough with magnets came in 1774. At that time, he had a female patient, Fraulein Oesterlin, who suffered from a variety of strange and chronic ailments. Mesmer decided to experiment with his new theory. He gave her a solution containing iron and placed magnets on her stomach and legs. She felt a mysterious fluid running throughout her body (similar perhaps to the sensation of *chi* reported by people having acupuncture), and her symptoms began to disappear. She continued with the treatment and recovered completely. From this one dramatic case, Mesmer's reputation was established.

As his popularity grew, however, controversy and scandal began to surround Mesmer, and in 1777 he left Vienna for Paris under a cloud. In Paris he set up a very successful practice in magnetic healing and wrote *Memoire sur la découverte du magnétisme animal (On the Discovery of Animal Magnetism)*, his text on magnets. In this work, Mesmer expanded on his hypothesis that there was a physical magnetic fluid that interconnects everything in the universe. He argued that disease was caused by an imbalance of this fluid within the body.

Mesmer claimed that the physician could act as a conduit for this animal magnetism and that this force could be channeled out of the universe and into the patient's body. Mesmer's theory is similar to that of the Chinese practice of Chi Gong and to modern ideas about energy healing. In common with modern concepts of electrical energy, with Wilhelm Reich's theory of orgone energy, and with Chinese ideas of chi, Mesmer saw magnetic fluid as something that was polarized, conductible, and able to be discharged and accumulated.[10]

While undergoing one of Mesmer's treatments, a patient would experience a magnetic "crisis," rather like an electric shock, after which the patient was cured. This phenomenon has a somewhat religious flavor. It sounds similar to the *shaktipat* of the Hindu tradition in which the devotee experiences a moment of shock that precedes a healing and awakening, or like the Evangelical spiritual healing practices in which the worshiper has a moment of unconsciousness before, for example, walking again.

To aid his treatments, Mesmer developed a device that he called the *baquet*, which concentrated magnetic fluid in a manner similar to a Leyden jar. With this contraption, Mesmer could treat twenty patients at once, each connected to the fluid via an iron rod.

In 1784, the King of France, Louis XVI, appointed a commission of scientists and physicians to investigate Mesmer's practices. The commission, which included Benjamin Franklin, reported that Mesmer was unable to support his claims with any scientific evidence, and, as a result, his popularity sharply declined. It remains a matter of conjecture whether they came to this conclusion because Mesmer was a complete charlatan, or whether it was because science was not developed enough to be able to explain what he was doing.

Like other medical pioneers who have worked with the concept of energy, such as Wilhelm Reich, Mesmer ended his days in obscurity, his discoveries discredited by the medical establishment. He died in 1815 in the small town close to his birthplace to which he had retired, his reputation shattered.[11] Despite his unfortunate end, he is remembered as the man who originated the modern theory of the unconscious and as the father of hypnosis.

EUROPE AFTER MESMER

Mesmer's ideas continued to be developed by other practitioners, most notably by Armand-Marie-Jacques de Chastenet, Marquis de Puységur (1751–1825). As early as 1784, Puységur recognized that both the patient's and the practitioner's belief, and the power of the relationship between the two, bore a significant impact on the success of the cure. The theories of

Puységur—considered by many as the founder of modern psychotherapy by merit of his experiments with hypnotism—are a fascinating prelude to today's scientific understanding of both the placebo effect and the Heisenberg principle, which states that the observer influences the experiment (see chapter 4).

Then came Jean-Martin Charcot (1825–1893), a successful physician and creator of the world's first neurology research center. Charcot came to believe that the physical phenomena that occurred during hypnosis could be transferred from one side of the body to the other by using magnets. When it became clear that this transfer occurred as part of the suggestibility of the hypnotic trance, Charcot's reputation was unfortunately tarnished.[12] Once again, a mistaken understanding of the nature of magnet therapy caused the end of a promising physician's career. Modern-day practitioners beware!

MAGNETS IN AMERICA

Throughout the nineteenth century and much of the twentieth century, magnet therapy in the United States was chiefly practiced by the kind of doctors who were derided as quacks by the discerning public and by the medical profession. Magnets were sold commercially and were advertised in widely available catalogs. In the late 1800s, the Sears catalog offered magnetic boot inserts for sale. Thatcher's Chicago Magnetic Company sold various magnetic caps and clothing by mail order.[13] Dr. Thatcher claimed (much as many magnet sellers do today) that "magnetism properly applied will cure every curable disease no matter what the cause."[14]

The number of people who actually used magnets in the late 1800s and early 1900s is not known. It is known, however, that the medical profession at that time was thoroughly against magnets. In the early 1900s,

Dr. Albert Abrams, a proponent of magnet therapy, was called the Dean of Twentieth-Century Charlatans by the American Medical Association.[15] But science was about to change this one-sided view, and beginning in the 1930s, researchers slowly began to amass some hard evidence about magnets and electromagnetic fields.

One of the earliest experiments took place in 1938. Dr. K. Hansen conducted a study using electromagnetic fields on patients suffering from conditions that had been diagnosed as sciatica, lumbago, and arthralgia. Out of 26 subjects, 23 reported rapid and significant relief of their pain. The study was not double-blinded (meaning that Dr. Hansen knew which patients were getting the placebo, although the patients did not), but there was no change reported by the two patients to whom the electromagnetic device was applied without the electricity being turned on.[16]

During the next thirty years, magnetism was little studied in the United States, although scientists in the Soviet Union, Japan, and Eastern Europe performed many studies. For various reasons, it was easier for scientists in those countries to get funding for research.

Informed by the Soviet research, some American scientists began to look at the therapeutic potential for electromagnetism, particularly for mending bone. Investigating electrical factors in bone and bone healing, U.S. scientists Robert Becker and Andrew Bassett showed as early as 1964 that broken bone had a higher than usual electrical current while it was healing. They also showed that in fractures that failed to heal, this naturally occurring electrical current was weak.

In 1971, Dr. Zachary Friedenberg of the University of Pennsylvania successfully used electrical treatment on a nonunion fracture in a human being. However, this technique involved surgical intervention, as the electrode had to be embedded directly into the bone marrow. Andrew Bassett, Arthur Pilla, and coworkers developed the use of a pulsed electromagnetic field in a noninvasive approach. In 1978, the FDA approved the use of this electromagnetic field therapy for the treatment of delayed or nonunion fractures.

It has been estimated that by 1986 more than 80 percent of orthopedic surgeons in the United States had used pulsed electromagnetic field therapy on at least one patient, with a success rate of 75 to 80 percent. The vast majority of treatment was for nonunion fractures, fusion failures, and pseudoarthrosis.[17] Since this breakthrough in orthopedic medicine, many more studies on the therapeutic use of magnetism have been undertaken. The vast majority of these studies have concerned pulsing electromagnetic fields, but in recent years some credible studies have demonstrated that permanent magnets also have a therapeutic effect.

Since the early 1970s, when electromagnetic machines made in Germany became available, U.S. sports medicine doctors have been interested in using magnets on injuries. Dr. Ernest Vandeweghe, doctor to the Los Angeles Lakers basketball team for fourteen years and a pediatrician at UCLA Medical School, was an early proponent of both electromagnetic and permanent magnet therapy and is now an adviser to the Nikken corporation. (Nikken is a large, multilevel Japanese marketing company that sells magnetic products.)

Of all sports professionals, golfers have been particularly keen to use magnets. This is probably because they tend to be a little older, and magnets seem to work effectively on conditions brought about by wear and tear. Prominent golfers such as Jim Colbert have done a good deal to promote the use of magnets on chronic injuries and general aches and pains. Veterinarians have also been among the early professional groups to embrace magnet therapy. In the past decade, the use of magnets on dogs and horses, particularly to speed the healing of injuries, has become increasingly widespread.

During the 1990s, magnets and magnetic products became more and more available to the American public. As a result, anecdotal evidence has begun to accrue, showing that magnets apparently stimulate healing in a variety of conditions. Since the mid-1990s, there has been an increase in the number of scientific studies designed to measure the effectiveness of magnetic therapy, which brings us to the present time. Before looking at how modern scientists are at last doing meaningful research into magnets, however, it is important to understand a little about what magnets actually do and why it is that they might have an effect on the physical body.

3

The Science of
Magnets and Magnetism

*"Magnetism is a dimly understood intrinsic property
of matter that manifests itself in two polarities."*

Robert Becker,
*The Body Electric: Electromagnetism
and the Foundation of Life*

Magnetism is fundamental to life. The magnetic field
protects the earth and allows life to flourish. Without
that field, the earth's atmosphere would not exist
because of constant bombardment by solar winds. The
crucial nature of magnetism makes it an area of scientific study that is both compelling and, in many ways,
still mysterious.

At a literal level, humankind's existence depends on
the earth's magnetic field. At a symbolic level, human
life itself continues because of the power of attraction
between men and women. Falling in love involves a
sense of being magnetized to the loved one in a way that
can bypass reason, just as disaffection can cause a sense
of repulsion that is equally insistent. Magnetism is the
most basic of forces, and it can both attract and repel.

The search to understand and manipulate magnetic energy has led many physicians and scientists,
past and present, into controversial realms that have

threatened their careers and even their sanity. This search has also led scientists to claim that they understand the magnetic force and its effect on the body and to either decry or exaggerate the powers of magnets in healing. In fact, regardless of what these scientists say, there is still much to be known.

It is hardly surprising that when I looked up magnets and magnetism in various scientific reference books I got quite confused. Some sources said that the only type of magnet found naturally was lodestone. Others said that magnetite and iron ore were both natural magnets, implying that they were two different things. Some books said that lodestone was a particular kind of magnetite, while others said that lodestone was an equivalent term for magnetite. Some sources said that the earth's magnetic field was decreasing, while others said that it was stable. Some references defined the north-polarized side of a magnet as that which was attracted to the North Pole, whereas others defined the north side as that which was repelled by the North Pole.

How could there be so much disagreement over magnets and magnetism? After all, they are a commonly occurring phenomena of nature and have been investigated since the dawn of science. What is more, magnetism is so pervasive that the very existence of life on the planet depends upon it.

I asked a geophysicist from the United States Geological Survey (USGS) if he would help explain all this contradiction and confusion to me. What he told me helped me understand why all the books were so confusing. As usual, the truth turns out to be both simpler and a little more complex. With many thanks to the authors whom I read and the scientists whom I questioned, what follows is, I hope, a clear and accurate explanation of the basic science of magnets and magnetism. If you find some of this challenging to understand, please bear in mind that electricity and magnetism is one of the toughest college courses and that there are fewer doctorates given in electrical engineering than in any of the other major science disciplines.

WHAT IS MAGNETISM?

Magnetism is a force that either attracts or repels. Certain objects exert magnetism on one another, even when they are not in contact. Objects that can act at a distance in this way are called magnets or are said to be magnetized. For example, if you put a paper clip an inch away from a magnet, the paper clip will be pulled toward the magnet and stick to its side. In this instance, the paper clip is magnetized.

WHAT IS A MAGNETIC FIELD?

A magnetic field is the area over which the magnetic force is exerted. If an attractable object comes into the magnetic field of the magnet, that object will be pulled toward the magnet.

WHAT IS A MAGNET?

Magnets can occur naturally or can be made by human beings. Anything that has electrons that can be aligned can be magnetized. What this means is, if you heat a substance or apply an electric current to it and then place it in the magnetic field of a magnet, the substance will take up the magnetic charge of the magnet. The electrons of the substance will realign themselves in lines that are organized in direction by polar north and south. Not all substances contain electrons that can be aligned. Iron is particularly amenable to alignment.

WHAT IS A NATURAL MAGNET?

Natural magnets are minerals that can hold a magnetic field. Such minerals are called ferrous metals, and they include iron (Fe), cobalt (Co), and nickel (Ni). Humankind has used iron since prehistoric times. According to the book of Genesis, the first book of the Bible, Tubal-Cain, seven generations from Adam, was "an instructor of every artificer in brass and iron." Smelted iron artifacts have been identified from around 3000 B.C.E.

The most common ferrous metal is magnetite, which is a form of iron. The common name for magnetite is lodestone. There is a good deal of lodestone on the planet. Lodestone is common enough that ancient peoples would have had relatively easy access to it. The largest magnetite deposits are found in northern Sweden.

There are also huge pieces of rock that contain large amounts of magnetite, such as those found in Death Valley. Some of these rocks are as big as a medium-sized room and have a magnetism that is strong enough to put nearby compasses and measuring equipment out of alignment.

How Are Natural Magnets Formed?

Magnets are formed as by-products of volcanic activity. When a volcano erupts, molten lava comes up out of the earth. This lava is predominately made up of iron, and some of this iron is in the form of magnetite. When the lava cools, the magnetite within takes on the magnetic characteristics of the earth's magnetic field. When the magnetite cools below a critical temperature, called the Curie Point, it becomes magnetic.

Magnetite is a mineral, and, like all minerals, it has a unique crystal structure. It is the crystal structure of magnetite that causes the magnetism. When the magnetite in the lava cools and changes from a liquid to a solid, magnetite crystals form.

Magnetite is made up of two forms of iron—iron +3 and iron +2. This means that the electrical charges on iron +3 differ from those on iron +2. These two differently charged types of iron occupy specific locations in the crystal structure of magnetite. This arrangement causes a transfer of electrons between the two different irons in a structured path, or vector. This electric vector inside the magnetite generates the magnetic field.

COULD ANCIENT CIVILIZATIONS HAVE MADE MAGNETS?

Definitely. It's not difficult to make a magnet out of iron. All you need is fire, a piece of lodestone (magnetite), and a piece of iron. Just like lava when it comes out of the earth, red-hot iron can be magnetized under the right conditions. When you forge a piece of iron until it is red hot and then place it right next to a piece of lodestone, the iron will take on the magnetic properties of the lodestone as it cools. When the iron is not totally solid but has been made plastic by the application of intense heat, the electrons within the structure of the metal are susceptible to being arranged into lines, thus creating a magnetic field. The closer to liquid a substance is, the easier the electrons in it can move about.

A regular piece of iron contains little regions, called domains, which are scrambled randomly throughout the iron. When the iron is magnetized, these domains line up and point in the same direction. The direction in which they point is north at one end and south at the other. And that is how a magnet is made.

Even the static electricity generated simply by rubbing certain substances can create a magnetic field.

There are references to ancient peoples rubbing amber to magnetize it and use it for healing purposes. In 600 B.C.E., the Greek philosopher, mathematician, and astronomer Thales observed that when a piece of amber is rubbed on clothing, the amber will attract or repel lightweight objects near it.

Likewise, you can rub a needle with a magnet to make a compass that can measure magnetic north. Simply rubbing the needle with the magnet will create enough friction—and therefore heat—to cause the atoms in the needle to line up, and so it becomes magnetized. Float the magnetized needle on water, and it will float around to magnetic north.

THE EARTH'S MAGNETIC FIELD

The earth acts like a huge, spherical magnet. It is surrounded by a magnetic field that is produced by the planet itself. The earth's magnetic field is like the field of a dipole magnet (a magnet with a north and south pole), with the magnet situated in the center of the earth.

What creates the earth's magnetic field? The earth is rotating all the time. This rotation, combined with extreme changes in temperature, causes the viscous fluids deep within the earth to move by a process known as convection. The magma in the core of the earth is made up of sludgy, molten iron, which is hotter in the center because of the pressure from gravity. This pressure and heat make the molten iron less dense, or lighter, and it very, very gradually moves toward the surface. The cooler molten iron closer to the earth's crust has a higher density, so it is heavier and very, very gradually begins to sink toward the center of the earth. These movements create a circular flow of iron that, because iron is charged, generates an electrical field that, in turn, generates the earth's protective magnetic field.

You can think of the convection within the earth as being similar to a water boiling in a pot. The heated water at the bottom of the pot rises to the top, while the cooler, heavier water at the top sinks toward the bottom. When you stop boiling the water, it slowly cools until everything reaches the same temperature and the convection process (which causes movement) stops. When the water is all at the same temperature and has stopped moving, it has reached a state of equilibrium. In the context of a planet, the convection process takes hundreds of millions of years to reach equilibrium. The earth is a long way from that stage. Other planets, however, have reached equilibrium. For example, Mars has achieved internal equilibrium, which is why it does not have a magnetic field. Loss of this magnetic field has allowed Mars to be bombarded by solar winds for hundreds of millions of years. These solar winds blew the Martian atmosphere away into space, which is why it is unlikely that there is life on Mars.

The dynamic relationship between the inner core and outer mantle of the earth creates the earth's magnetic field, thus allowing life to flourish. Magnetism is about dynamic equilibrium; so we can also say that life itself is dependent on the attraction of opposites.

Is the Earth's Magnetic Field Changing?

Some proponents of magnet therapy claim that we need it in order to increase our exposure to natural magnetic energy. In 1976, Dr. Kyoichi Nakagawa, a prominent Japanese doctor, proposed that many modern-day ailments were caused by a condition that he termed Magnetic Field Deficiency Syndrome (MFDS). According to this theory, MFDS gives rise to a syndrome similar to chronic fatigue and fibromyalgia, and these disorders may in fact be caused by MFDS. Some alternative practitioners in the West have picked up this idea, and many Web sites and magnet sellers now claim that many people are suffering from MFDS. To back up this assertion, adherents of this theory claim that the earth's magnetic field is decreasing at a rate that affects the vitality of life on the planet. Some of these sources cite official-sounding data that, on the surface, seem convincing. However, this information is misleading.

As mentioned earlier, the earth is constantly rotating. This rotation, combined with the convection of matter within the earth, creates a dynamic effect in which the earth's outside shell affects the inside core and the inside core affects the outside shell. As a result of all this activity, the magnetic field is continually changing.

There are horizontal and vertical components to the earth's magnetic field. Due to the rotational forces of the earth, the field is generally aligned with the earth's geographic poles. This means that there is a north and south, or vertical, magnetic field. There is also a circulating force, or the horizontal magnetic field.[1] The compass measures the horizontal magnetic field, which is changing all the time because the continents are shifting. Now, if we only consider the horizontal magnetic field, then yes, at times, it does seem that the earth's magnetic field is decreasing. However, as I've shown, the horizontal is only one component of the entire magnetic field of the earth.

The National Geomagnetic Information Center at the USGS says that the magnetic field *is* decreasing, but very slowly and not at all at the rate claimed by the proponents of the diminishing magnetic field theory. The dipolar magnetic field, which constitutes 90 percent of the earth's total magnetic field, remained virtually unchanged throughout the twentieth century. The nondipole field, which constitutes the other 10 percent, "fluctuates significantly over decade time scales, apparently reflecting the unsteady exchange of angular momentum between the core and the mantle."[2]

Because the earth's magnetic field is constantly changing, it is impossible to predict what the field will be in the distant future. In addition, there are significant regional variations in the strength of the magnetic field. According to the geophysicist at the USGS, "If you look at a geomagnetic map, you will see that the earth's magnetic field varies enormously from place to place. To say that, in general, we're suffering from this magnetic field deficiency doesn't seem reasonable."

Another factor cited by some magnet therapy proponents as being a causative factor in MFDS is that, because of modern technology, we are constantly exposed to magnetic fields. The theory goes that this exposure has a negative influence on our ability to tap into the earth's natural electromagnetic field.

Just to clarify this issue: the electromagnetic fields we create are not changing the earth's electromagnetic fields, although they may still affect our health. In addition, there is no evidence to verify the idea that human-made electromagnetic fields interfere with our capacity to absorb the earth's magnetic field. There has been a good deal of research into the negative effects of electromagnetic fields, with no clear, irrefutable data yet, either way.

POWER SPOTS: DO SOME PLACES HAVE MORE MAGNETIC ENERGY THAN OTHERS?

Some areas of the earth have a higher magnetic charge than other areas have, because of the rock in that region. When magma cools and changes from a liquid to a solid, the magnetite within it takes on the magnetic field of the earth at the time that the lava cools. As we've already seen, the earth's magnetic field fluctuates in intensity over time, so rock takes on the magnetic characteristics of the earth at the time it solidified. How magnetite forms depends on the rate at which the magma cools. It's like making good toffee. If you cook the toffee too fast, it burns. If you don't get it hot enough, the toffee won't solidify properly. Similarly, the cooling process of lava segregates various minerals, producing veins of gold and other metals in the earth's crust.

Over geologic time, powdered magnetite that erodes from lava washes into the streams, then settles into lakes and creates varved clays—or clays that have thin layers of magnetite within them. Scientists can measure these varves to determine what the earth's magnetic field was long ago. Scientists have flown over the land with magnetometers (instruments for measuring the earth's magnetic field), and they have towed magnetometers behind boats at sea. Using these techniques, scientists have been able to map the variations in the earth's magnetic field over geologic time. These magnetic signatures of a certain region of the planet enable us to understand how the landmasses have moved around.

There are certain spots on the earth that many people experience as powerful, such as Sedona, Arizona, and Lourdes, France. It may be that these places have stronger magnetic fields than other areas, although I could find no data to support this idea. Another thought that occurred to me as I was researching this particular aspect of magnetism was whether the great civilizations developed in areas that had a particularly strong magnetic field at that time. This is a question for further study.

DO MAGNETS HELP ASTRONAUTS STAY HEALTHY IN OUTER SPACE?

Another common magnet myth is a persistent story about astronauts and the early space missions. This tale turns up on numerous Web pages, in various books, and at lectures given by proponents of magnet therapy. According to the story, when the astronauts came back from space travel severely debilitated, someone at NASA realized that their exhaustion was due to having been outside the earth's magnetic field. As a remedy, in future space trips, magnets were placed inside the astronauts' spacesuits or in a big dome at the top of the spacecraft, depending on which version of the story you hear. This story has been used to support the notion that magnetism is essential for human health. Well, no one is disputing that—as we've seen, human life would not exist without the earth's magnetic field. But is this outer space story true?

When I asked the geophysicist from the USGS about this story, he said, "I was involved in several of the Gemini space missions, and I never heard anything about this. And, anyway, magnets might interfere with other electronic and navigational equipment of the spacecraft." Then I read on a NASA Web page that spaceships are degaussed (i.e., demagnetized) before leaving the earth's atmosphere so as not to interfere with the instrumentation of the ship. I called NASA and their spokesman told me that he had never heard of magnets being added to spacesuits or anywhere else to help the astronauts. As with the other experts I consulted, he also agreed that such an idea made no scientific sense.

It is undoubtedly true that the earth's magnetic field has a crucial influence on the health of the living beings dwelling on the planet. It may also be true that astronauts suffer as a result of being out of this magnetic field for a period of time. But it is entirely illogical to jump to the conclusion that this means we all need extra doses of magnetism in order to be healthy.

HOW ARE MAGNETS MANUFACTURED?

As we have already seen, it's not difficult to make a magnet out of any form of iron, as long as you have a piece of already magnetized rock. By the end of the nineteenth century, all the known elements and many compounds had been tested for magnetism, and only three elements—iron, nickel, and cobalt—were found to be amenable to being permanently magnetized.

Magnets today are mostly ceramic magnets, which means that they are made out of iron filings and clay baked together. During this baking process, the ceramic is subjected to a very strong DC magnetic current field. This artificially recreates what happens in the earth when magnetite, or lodestone, is made by combining the intense heat of molten lava with the earth's own magnetic field. The difference is that at the earth's surface, the magnetic field is relatively weak—at the most, about 2 to 3 gauss and, on average, about 0.5 gauss. Today, magnets are made that measure in the thousands of gauss. The strength of a magnet depends on how much iron is in it, its shape, and what level of magnetism it is exposed to. Just as the amount of iron is a factor in the strength of a magnet, the size and weight of a magnet can be an indicator of its strength.

Unlike lodestone, which has a random, lumpy shape, certain geometric shapes—for example, round and flat with a hole in the center—take on more gauss than others do. Steel magnets in the form of bars, horseshoes, and U-shapes are used mainly in science education. Neodymium rare earth magnets are used for education, industry, and magic. They are also used as therapeutic magnets. Ferrites are low-cost alternatives to neodymium.

WHAT IS ELECTROMAGNETISM?

Electricity and magnetism are bound together. When an electrical current flows in a wire, the movement of the electrons through the wire produces a magnetic field in the space around the wire. In the case of a direct current

(DC), the current flows in one direction and the magnetic field is steady.

If the current is fluctuating (also called pulsing or pulsating), the magnetic field is also fluctuating. An example of a fluctuating current is an alternating current (AC), which switches directions all the time. The strength of the magnetic field depends upon the amount of electricity flowing through the wire. The more current, the stronger the magnetic field produced. A fluctuating magnetic or electromagnetic field is measured by its rate of fluctuation. One fluctuation per second equals one hertz.

Fields produced by electricity and magnetism are described as electrical, magnetic, or electromagnetic. These terms are distinguished from one another as follows: an electrical field is predominately electrical; there's no actual magnet, just the magnetic field always produced by current. With a magnetic field, there is a magnet but no electrical current, other than the slight electrical charge that may be produced by the action of magnetism. With an electromagnetic field, an electric current is passed through or around a magnet, which amplifies the effects of both qualities of energy.

An electrical current always produces both an electric and a magnetic field, the strength of which depends on the configuration of wires in which the current is flowing. A wire coil, such as in a transformer, produces a significantly larger magnetic field than a single strand of wire. A time-varying magnetic field also induces an electric field. A static magnet does not induce an electric field.

MEASURING THE STRENGTH OF MAGNETS

The strength of permanent magnets is measured in gauss and tesla. There are 10,000 gauss to 1 tesla.

Therapeutic magnets are measured in gauss. A refrigerator magnet measures approximately 50 to 100 gauss at the surface and 200 gauss at the center of the magnet. The most commonly used therapeutic magnets range from 50 to 2,000 gauss at the surface. The manufacturer's rating of the magnet will often be higher than this, usually indicating the gauss of the magnet at its strongest place, that is, in the center of the magnet. Sometimes the manufacturer will specify whether the given rating applies to the surface of the magnet.

As you might imagine, magnetic field weakens the further you are from the surface of the magnet. When you put a magnet on your body, the amount of magnetism received by the target tissue depends on how far the tissue is from the magnet. When treating an acupuncture point or a condition that is very close to the body surface, such as a wrist sprain, the surface field measurement of the magnet is fairly close to the dose that the person is receiving. But when treating a pain in the deep muscles of the back, the magnetic dose may be much lower than the magnet surface rating. Also, as mentioned earlier, the strength of a magnet is related to its size. The strength of small magnets decays much more rapidly with distance than that of large magnets.

POLARITIES

All magnets have a north-seeking pole and a south-seeking pole. In magnet circles, controversy rages about polarity. There has been much confusion about which side of the magnet is named north. Traditional science calls the north side of the magnet the side *attracted* to the earth's North Pole—that is, the north side is the north-seeking pole.

In the early development of magnet therapy, this naming convention somehow got reversed, and the north pole of the magnet was named as the side *repelled* by the earth's North Pole—that is, the south-seeking pole. This means that the magnet has the same polarity as the earth's north magnetic pole. So in magnet therapy, the north pole of a magnet is the south-seeking pole and registers negative on a gauss meter (−). The south pole is the north-seeking pole and registers positive on a gauss meter (+).

In addition to this confusion, there is disagreement about how to use polarities in treatment. Some practitioners consider that the success of certain therapies depends on whether you have the north or the south polarity facing the skin. This choice depends on the nature of the condition being treated. Others say that it is more effective to use both poles at the same time in an alternating-pole configuration. No one knows the definitive answer to this question, although opinions on the matter are strong. (For more detailed discussion, see chapter 11.)

MEDICAL USES OF MAGNETISM

Probably the best known use of magnetism in medicine is magnetic resonance imaging (MRI). The MRI was developed by several teams of scientists in the 1970s. One of these scientists was the biophysicist Dr. Carlton Hazlewood, who, two decades later, designed the Baylor Study, which showed that magnets help relieve pain (see chapter 5).

An MRI delivers a huge blast of magnetic energy, utilizing magnetic fields in the range of 1.5 to 2.5 tesla (15,000–25,000 gauss). Any matter that has electrons can be excited by a magnetic field. The MRI then reads how the resonance calms itself back down. In order to calm itself back down, the resonance has to radiate back out another electrical field. The MRI reads that process.

Geophysicists use the MRI to see inside the earth, in the same way that doctors use the MRI to see what is happening inside living bodies.

Interestingly, there have been reports of people with Parkinson's disease having no movement problems for 24 hours after having an MRI and of people with Alzheimer's being completely lucid for a similar period of time. These reports suggest that a powerful magnetic field can somehow reorganize brain activity. Researchers are integrating these accidental findings into their studies on these two debilitating diseases.

Magnetic technology is also proving to be helpful in other areas of medicine. In 1998, the first magnetically controlled brain surgery was carried out at the Washington University School of Medicine in St. Louis, Missouri. This exciting new development combines magnetic devices of two types: the magnetic control of surgical tools and the magnetic resonance imaging scan technique. In the operation, a catheter was moved through a patient's brain by superconducting magnets to take a biopsy of a tumor. A surgeon using a computer mouse directed the path taken by the catheter. The magnetic fields on the tip of the catheter allowed the surgeon to guide surgical instruments along a curved path through the brain with far greater navigational control. Previously, surgical instruments have had to take a straight-line path to the target, creating more risk of damaging other tissue.[3]

THE BODY AND MAGNETISM

The body creates electrical currents that, in turn, generate magnetic fields. The heart and the brain are particularly active electrically. It is now known that there is a magnetic substance, known as biogenic magnetite (a biologically created form of magnetite), in the brain, heart, spleen, and liver. This substance may also exist in other parts of the body.

A recent and ongoing collaborative research project among scientists in Switzerland, Hawaii, and Australia has shown that the human brain contains biogenic magnetite. This finding is important because it means that there may be a mechanism by which environmental magnetic fields interact with the central nervous system, although this is highly controversial at present. The team of researchers continues to work together to understand how amounts of biogenic magnetite may influence brain disorders, such as epilepsy.[4]

At present, the function of this biogenic magnetite in the brain is not clearly understood. Some of the same researchers in Switzerland and Australia are also investigating the magnetic properties of the heart, spleen, and liver. Their research indicates that there are ferrimagnetic, fine-grained, magnetically interacting particles in these organs—new evidence that there is biogenic magnetite in organs other than the brain. According to the researchers, "This material probably is not used for geomagnetic-field sensing in humans. It may represent an extra iron dump for the body, or clusters of magnetite particles could be a site of magnetochemistry. At this point, however, the role of the magnetite in humans is unknown."[5] Although we don't know what all this means, a picture of the human body as a biomagnetic organism, as well as a biochemical and biophysical entity, is beginning to emerge.

A PERSPECTIVE ON ELECTROMAGNETICS

David Levy, creator of the trackball and much of the Macintosh® PowerBook® computer, is now an independent inventor who has done a study on the processes of invention. Discussing inventing methods, he said,

"You could go down . . . the list of physical implementations: mechanical, thermal, chemical, electronic, and electromagnetic. Generally, products start out mechanical and end up electromagnetic."[6] This puts in perspective the place of electromagnetics in modern medicine. Of course, we don't know what will come after electromagnetics, if anything. For now, the electromagnetic method of energy delivery is the most advanced we have to offer.

WHAT IS BIOELECTROMAGNETICS?

Bioelectromagnetics is an emerging scientific discipline. It studies how living organisms interact with electromagnetic fields. The body produces electrical currents that create magnetic fields that extend outside the body. These fields can be affected by external fields and currents. This interrelationship may create changes in the natural fields of the body, with physical and behavioral consequences, both positive and negative.

At this time, bioelectromagnetics has two main areas of interest. The first is the possible harmful effect of electromagnetic fields on human health from such things as power lines. The second is the study of the healing potential of low-frequency electromagnetic fields.

SUMMARY

In this chapter, I have merely scratched the surface of the science of magnets and magnetism. As you can imagine, lengthy tomes are written on this subject alone. What I have endeavored to give you in this chapter are some basic definitions—some building blocks— to help you understand the place of magnets and magnetism in the overall scheme of things. This information should also help you understand how magnets are being used, researched, and fantasized about in medicine today. In addition, you should now know enough to be able to distinguish some of the truths from falsehoods that occur in the world of magnets.

In the next six chapters, we look at the current state of research on magnets, beginning with a general overview of the politics and prevailing paradigm of modern medical research, and then looking specifically at how this affects our knowledge of magnet therapy.

Part 2

Scientific Research

4

Scientific Research on Magnet Therapy

Research into the therapeutic use of magnets is a relatively recent field of study in the United States and Western Europe. It has only been in the past few years that doctors and scientists have begun to take magnets seriously as a method of healing. However, in other parts of the world, the situation has been different. The therapeutic uses of magnets and electromagnetism have been investigated far more in Eastern Europe, the former Soviet Union, and some parts of Asia than they have in the United States or in Western Europe. There are several reasons for this difference.

In the Western world, medical science in the twentieth century was dominated by biochemistry. The West continues to be influenced by the fundamental concept that healing occurs by influencing blood chemistry. When chemical means fail, the remedy of next resort is surgery.

Physics, the science of matter and energy and the interaction between the two in a number of fields, including electricity and magnetism, gives rise to a discipline known as biophysics—the physics of the body. During the twentieth century—despite the introduction of x-rays and MRIs—biophysics has been secondary to biochemistry, in overall terms and certainly in terms of fundamental thinking. This situation developed due to certain key factors in the development of modern medicine.

Until the early twentieth century, a great deal of medical care included remedies that sprang from our understanding of biophysics, such as the application of heat and cold. However, in the 1930s and 1940s, the breakthrough remedies of sulfur and antibiotic drugs revolutionized medical care. All of a sudden, it was possible to cure infectious disease by taking a pill. The new drugs were so wonderfully effective that they caused a seismic shift in health care. Both medical practitioners and patients became more focused on pills as the primary way for medicine to be delivered. This trend meant that more and more money went toward pharmaceutical manufacturers, who in turn put more and more money into drug research and had more and more reason to focus health concerns on the idea of "magical" pills.

In eastern Europe and Asia, for a combination of cultural and economic reasons, medical thinking developed somewhat differently. In such places as China, Russia, and Japan, there already existed a powerful tradition of biophysical health care, including acupuncture, various kinds of massage, martial arts, hydrotherapy, and magnet therapy. In addition, in these countries, particularly in the Communist countries and in post–World War II Japan, finances were more restricted. Neither patients nor governments could afford to favor exclusively the use of expensive new drugs from the West. Therefore there was considerable interest in developing cheaper methods of health-care delivery, which is why acupuncture flourished under Maoist China. Mao certainly supported bringing back acupuncture as another traditional Chinese practice, but its renewal was also due to its healing effectiveness.

The Chinese are, above all, pragmatists. By figuring out which aspects of acupuncture and other methods of traditional Chinese medicine were really effective, they were able to create a cost-efficient and simple health-care system. They encouraged and financed scientific studies into traditional Chinese healing techniques. These studies resulted in many changes in medical practice, such as the routine use of acupuncture as anesthesia in Cesarean sections, as well as massive changes in the health care available to poor people, whom, in China, as in most of the world, were the vast majority of the population.

During the 1960s, the Chinese developed the concept of the "Barefoot Doctor." Thousands of people were taught simple herbal and acupuncture formulas and basic first aid and were sent out into rural areas to provide free or very inexpensive medical care. This concept, born of necessity and combined with a desire for cultural betterment, fueled interest in magnets as another cheap and relatively easy form of treatment. A southern Chinese lineage had used magnets for several centuries. Medical practitioners from other parts of China, from Japan, and from other countries came to southern China to study magnet therapy from the teachers of this lineage.

The technically minded Japanese took to magnet therapy with enthusiasm. Their technical background, coupled with the natural affinity between acupuncture and magnet therapy (acupuncture was already very popular in Japan), influenced Japanese practitioners, most notably Yoshio Manaka. (Chapter 12 covers this subject in greater depth.)

In the former Soviet Union, both doctors and the government were eager to explore methods of healing that did not rely on relatively expensive biochemical means. In southern Russia, one ethnic group was discovered to be using magnetic rocks (lodestone) around broken bones. This practice was one of the stimuli that began the Russian exploration into magnet therapy. In the Soviet Union and eastern Europe, many studies on magnetic and electromagnetic therapy were undertaken.

The fall of the Berlin Wall in 1989 and the subsequent break up of the Soviet Union wreaked havoc with scientific research in that part of the world, and much government funding was withdrawn. Many eastern European doctors and scientists moved to the West to continue their research. Some of these men and women are currently influencing and informing research into magnetic therapies in the United States. One such scientist is Dr. Marko Markov, a Bulgarian biophysicist, who has been studying the effects of magnetic fields on living systems since 1969 and who is now affiliated with the Department of Orthopedics at Mount Sinai School of Medicine. He also works as a consultant to EMF Therapeutics, a company doing cutting-edge research into magnet therapy.

It has only been within the past few years that doctors and patients, en masse, have begun to understand the limits of chemical medicine. The reality of side effects—especially from the long-term use of drugs such as painkillers—has become all too clear. Consequently, there is growing interest in physical remedies. The inadequacies and limits of drug therapy are creating room for nonchemical remedies to enter the medical arena. During the past two decades, Americans have begun to embrace acupuncture, homeopathy, and the medicinal use of herbs. They are now looking at magnets as an alternative to pain-relieving medication.

RESEARCH INTO MAGNETS

Many studies have taken place on magnets outside the United States. For example, a Korean study on using magnets to help menstrual pain, several Japanese studies on magnetic mattress pads and magnetic bracelets, and a number of Russian and eastern European studies have taken place. The United States has lagged behind in interest in magnets for reasons already mentioned—the success of pharmaceutical and surgical remedies, physician bias, and various cultural factors.

In recent years, however, several credible studies on permanent magnets have been completed in the United States. The most notable of these are the Baylor Study on pain in post-polio syndrome (see chapter 5), Dr. Agatha Colbert's study on fibromyalgia (see chapter 6), Dr. Daniel Man's study on healing after liposuction surgery (see chapter 7), and Dr. Michael Weintraub's study on peripheral neuropathy (see chapter 8). But these studies can only be considered to be pilot studies, because none of them has involved more than 50 people.

Despite the fact that for several years magnets have been known to have an effect on pain, no decent, large-scale study has yet to be funded in the United States. The success of the pilot studies has not yet led to studies of a significant size. Why? Most likely it is because many people in the scientific and medical communities still think magnet therapy is, at best, a minor contribution to health care. The implications of the small studies have not yet filtered out to the majority of doctors and researchers in the field.

Until at least one large-scale study is completed in the United States, the Food and Drug Administration (FDA) is unlikely to give magnets full sanction as therapeutic devices. The FDA does not consider foreign medical studies to be valid. This limits the actions of both doctors and magnet marketers in terms of referrals, research, and advertising claims. The consumer is protected from some of the worst of excessive claims for magnets, although given the eternal quest for universal panaceae, these claims cannot entirely be policed out of existence (see Appendix: Magnets and the Law). The downside of the FDA's caution is that magnet therapy, a potentially useful technique, has been very slow to be implemented in medical care.

MAGNETS AND RESEARCH FUNDING

Pharmaceuticals currently dominate both the market-place and the philosophy and practice of medicine. Pharmaceutical companies are the main source of funds for medical research. It is not in their interests to put their money into magnet research and other nondrug therapies. Consequently, far less money is available for research of therapies such as magnets, acupuncture, and homeopathy than is available for the study of drug treatments. At the moment, most research into the use of static, or permanent, magnets is being done out of curiosity by physicians. For example, the Baylor Study (see chapter 5) was a volunteer effort on the part of the doctors, and the magnets were provided gratis by BIOflex®, a magnet manufacturer. For magnets to attract sufficient funding to do large-scale, thorough research, more pilot studies need to be completed.

SPECIAL RESEARCH ISSUES FOR MAGNETS

The placebo effect is easier to factor into a study when you are giving someone a pill than when you are using a manual therapy. With magnets there is a real danger of placebo detection. A subject in an experiment with magnets can always test the device with a paper clip to see if it is really magnetic. Although studies are policed to prevent this, it is still a potential problem.

And then there is the Heisenberg principle, which shows us that the beliefs of the people conducting the experiment have an effect upon the outcome. For this reason, scientists developed the double-blind trial, so that the clinicians are as blind to the nature of the devices as the subjects are. The double-blind format prevents subjects from receiving subliminal clues given by clinical personnel. There is also an effect beyond all of this, in which the beliefs and attitudes of the observers of an experiment affect the outcome.

Robert Jahn and Brenda Dunn, of the Princeton Engineering Anomalies Research Laboratory, have shown that people can skew the numbers on a random number generator simply by wishing the numbers to be high or low. These studies have shown that mental intention can interact with random physical systems. The studies suggest that scientists with a background belief that magnets work are more likely to produce results that show magnets work, compared with results derived from skeptical or seemingly neutral investigators. Such possibilities jeopardize the whole paradigm of objectivity upon which science currently rests. They also make it more difficult for new ideas to find acceptance, because repeat trials done by people who are skeptical are unlikely to turn up such good results as studies done by researchers with a positive attitude.

THE INFLUENCE OF THE MARKETPLACE

The only organizations currently driving the introduction of magnets in North America with any force are marketing companies. Many of these companies operate as multilevel marketing organizations, with the products sold by individual distributors rather than marketed directly or through wholesalers and retailers. Other companies are actively selling magnets via the Internet.

Why don't these magnet manufacturers fund good research, in the same way that the pharmaceutical companies do? Nikken, the largest of the multilevel marketing companies (global sales of $1.5 billion and 200 million customers worldwide), claims to have done its own research and to have concluded that devices with alternating polar fields are highly effective for reducing pain and inflammation and for enhancing sound sleep.

Yet, because of the FDA's current stand on magnets, Nikken's representatives say the company does not dare make public any of these findings. The company fears that it will be shut out of the lucrative U.S. market for making health-related claims for magnets. On the one hand, this sounds like fudging, and one is tempted to say that it is easy to claim to have done the studies, but that a big federal agency won't let that information be made public. Failing to disclose the results of the studies is a big disadvantage for the consumer and physician alike, who are deprived of knowing the results of the Nikken research (if such results are indeed both credible and favorable). But, on the other hand, Nikken says that it doesn't want to deprive Americans of the value of their products, which they would risk doing if they went public with the details of their research. Although once again, this sounds like a glib piece of marketing, Nikken products do occupy the high end of the magnet market, with some of the most sophisticated and well-constructed devices available for the lay person. Proponents of the company are convinced that the company's focus on wellness is a genuine service to humanity.

Whatever the reality—and it may include a mission for creating wellness as well as for creating corporate wealth—consumer demand for magnets far outstrips scientific research. This imbalance is gradually being corrected as credible studies get under way, fueled by the need to understand whether magnets can help pain and suffering and how this therapeutic effect occurs.

WHO IS DOING STUDIES INTO MAGNETS?

There are four main categories of researchers who are investigating the therapeutic value of magnets.

1. **The Biophysicists.** These are scientists who are investigating the effects of magnetism on the body. Usually they are involved with studying the effects of electromagnetism rather than the effects of static magnets (although recently some researchers have begun to explore the effects of static magnets). Some biophysicists, such as Dr. Arthur Pilla, at the Mount Sinai School of Medicine in New York, are attached to medical schools. Some are full-time consultants to magnet manufacturers, such as Dr. Marko Markov. Most prominent biophysicists serve as consultants to magnet manufacturers, even if they hold a full-time staff position at a university or medical school.

2. **The Inventors.** The inventors are also scientists who may or may not be attached to educational institutions and who have patented magnetic devices. Examples are Dr. Arthur Pilla, inventor of the Biosteogen, the first FDA-approved pulsed electromagnetic device for healing non- and delayed-union bone fractures; Dr. Richard Markoll, inventor of the Pulsed Signal Therapy device; and Dr. Jerry Jacobson, inventor of the Jacobson Resonator Unit. Markoll and Jacobson are both currently seeking FDA approval for their devices. There are also many other people experimenting with inventing magnetic and electromagnetic devices.

   The inventors in this field run the gamut from conscientious doctors and physicists to scientific mavericks whose inventions may even be dangerous. The inventors are sometimes funded privately by investors or by funds earned from using magnetic devices in countries in which their use is legal.

3. **The Physicians.** These are doctors, practicing conventional and/or alternative medicine, who want to know if magnets really work. They are usually

motivated to create research projects on magnets out of a desire to improve the range of the therapy they can offer their patients. Examples are Dr. Carlos Vallbona, a pediatrician who runs a pain clinic; Dr. Agatha Colbert, a physician/acupuncturist; Dr. Michael Weintraub, a neurologist; Dr. Daniel Man, a cosmetic surgeon; and Dr. Richard Rogachefsky, an orthopedic surgeon. To do studies, the physicians usually donate their time and ask manufacturers to give them magnets.

4. **Magnet Manufacturers.** These include companies that make static magnets and those that make electromagnetic devices. It is in the interests of the manufacturers to prove that magnets work and to find out the most efficacious ways of using them. As discussed above, many of the companies that sell magnets either have not performed significant research or have not published it. An exception is Magnetherapy, Inc., of Riviera Beach, Florida, which markets the Tectonic™ brand of magnetic devices. This company supported the studies performed by Dr. Colbert and Dr. Man, which are detailed in chapters 6 and 7, respectively.

Although Nikken claims to have performed extensive research, the company has not made this research public, for the reasons mentioned earlier. Many companies selling static magnets simply sell the products and cite other people's research in their literature, sometimes erroneously. Some of the more farsighted companies (mostly manufacturers of electromagnetic devices) are involved in cutting-edge research. For example, Magnetherapy is currently funding biophysical, cellular, and animal studies on dosage, strength, and effectiveness of static magnets; and EMF Therapeutics is currently experimenting on mice using electromagnetism to treat cancer by impeding blood flow to the tumor.

SCIENTIFIC STUDIES: WHY DO WE NEED THEM?

There are countless anecdotal reports that magnets are useful for treating pain and some other conditions. But are these reports enough? In today's world, no, they are not. In the past, the value of medical treatments was largely based on the experiences of doctors and patients. But as medicine has become more complex, we have learned that anecdotal evidence, although an important part of the picture, is too subjective to be reliable in every instance.

We now understand the placebo effect, which means that a treatment can gain effectiveness from the belief of the patient. Although this shows how powerfully our beliefs can affect the process of cure, it also means that the treatment may be unreliable and varying in its effectiveness from person to person. Today, people want to know with greater accuracy how well a treatment might work, regardless of the placebo effect. Society wants a finite and objective reality of medical care. No such reality can ever exist—people are too wonderfully variable for that to be possible—but perhaps the search to find it helps us understand health care and the human body with more precision.

There is also the crucial issue of side effects. Without scientific studies, we run the risk of finding out too late that a treatment has damaging side effects, long after many people have already used it. The reason we need regulatory institutions, like the FDA, is to avoid any more tragedies, such as that caused by thalidomide. The side effects of many modern medical treatments mean that we have to have a clear understanding of what they do to the body. For this kind of knowledge, a scientific study is essential.

Even magnets, benign as they might appear, need to be tested scientifically. Any form of medical intervention that is powerful has the potential to be damaging, and we need to understand under what circumstances damage might occur. Since we don't know how strong a magnet can be before it causes harm or what side effects there might be from sleeping on ultra-strong magnets night after night, studies are important and necessary.

WHAT MAKES A SCIENTIFIC STUDY VALID?

A good, valid study tells us if the treatment works, how to use it effectively, and if there are any side effects.

The first question to ask in determining whether a study is valid is whether the device or treatment is effective. Does it have a therapeutic action that can be measured by objective criteria?

The second question concerns the appropriate dosage and mode of applying the therapy. Is the dosage variable, or do the majority of people need the same dose given in the same way? Is dosage dependent on gender, age, body size, or type of ailment?

The third question concerns side effects. Is the treatment safe? Magnets, although apparently simple objects, may have an undesirable effect on some people in some circumstances. For example, we simply don't know if it is safe to use magnets during pregnancy; so, for safety's sake, most practitioners and salespeople recommend not using magnets during pregnancy. It is also possible, however, that magnets might be very helpful for the aches and pains of pregnancy, and they may be preferable to painkilling drugs. Studies would help find the answer to this and many other concerns.

The Four Criteria for a Valid Study

For a study to be valid, it needs to satisfy four criteria.

1. *The study must be repeatable,* meaning that another team of researchers in a different lab working with

different subjects should be able to get the same result.

2. *The study must be placebo-controlled,* meaning that there is a group of subjects in the experiment that doesn't receive any active therapy, but instead gets something that looks like the therapy, such as a sugar pill in a drug study or a fake magnet in a magnet study. The amount of positive response among the placebo group is measured against the number of subjects. If the therapy being examined has an effect beyond that of placebo, there will be a higher positive result in the real therapy group.

3. *The study should be double-blind,* meaning that neither the subjects nor the doctors or researchers know which patients are receiving the active therapy and which are getting the placebo. In a single-blind trial, the doctors know and the subjects don't. At one time it was thought that this single-blind approach was sufficient, until it became clear that doctors and nurses tend to communicate in subtle, often unconscious ways, with subjects whether the treatment is real or placebo. For the study to be clean, the blind must be double. If anyone in the study determines who is getting the placebo and who is getting the real thing, it is said that the blind has been broken, and the trial is no longer fully valid.

4. *The study sampling must be randomized,* meaning that a random selection process is used to decide who gets the active therapy and who gets the placebo. Randomized sampling helps to avoid bias in the results that might occur if the researchers were able to choose people for the real treatment whom they thought would do well.

The studies described in the following chapters meet some of these criteria. Some of the studies meet all of the criteria. None of the studies are sufficiently large to show overwhelming evidence for magnets, but they are valid studies that show promise. In addition to the group studies, some interesting case studies are included. A case study is the detailed record of a single case and is often used to gather funding for a larger study.

Which Studies to Believe?

When you hear of a scientific study, always look to see if it has been published in a professional, peer-reviewed journal. There are many studies on magnets that are reported on Web sites and elsewhere that are not credible scientifically, in the way we currently define *credibility*. Some studies are published in journals that seem credible, but that are in fact simply a mouthpiece for one author, such as Dr. William Philpott's *Magnetic Health Quarterly*. These studies may appear valid, but if they have not been published in a medical journal of repute, or at least presented at a genuine scientific conference, then you probably should not take them seriously.

Studies published in magazines and on Web sites devoted to magnets or presented at conferences run by magnet manufacturers should be looked at with some suspicion. When people tell you, "Oh, that's been proved scientifically," please don't take their word for it. Ask to see the data to back up their assertion. The world of magnet therapy is unfortunately rife with false scientific information. Better to hear, "Oh, we don't know how it works, but Auntie Mabel's hip is all better now," than to be conned into believing that there is objective evidence that simply does not exist.

With that caveat in mind, let's look at studies that have credibility and find out what they have to tell us about magnets. Chapters 5–8 detail several studies on the therapeutic use of permanent magnets. The book then looks at studies on electromagnetic field therapy.

5

Magnets and Pain
The Baylor Study

Annie and Sarah, whom we met in chapter 1, both suffered from pain. In Annie's case, the pain was chronic, meaning it was long lasting and resistant to treatment. The remedies offered to her by her doctors were to take painkilling drugs for the rest of her life or to have back surgery with no assured outcome. Instead, she tried magnets and was amazed to find that she experienced immediate relief. Within a few months of using the magnets, her long-term back pain went away almost completely.

Sarah suffered from acute pain, meaning that the pain was of recent origin. Her pain was caused by injuries sustained in a car accident. With an acute condition, because the body has not yet settled into a pattern, the prognosis for full recovery is usually better than for a chronic condition. With the proper treatment, complete recovery is possible. Sarah was offered pain medication by her doctor and told that her injuries would heal over time. True, she probably would have recovered on her own, but she couldn't afford to take a year getting well, missing work because of the medication's side effects. For her, painkillers were not an option, as they made her too fuzzyheaded to work. Magnets provided her with pain relief without side effects. As far as Sarah and her acupuncturist were concerned, magnets had the additional benefit of speeding up the healing process.

Like Sarah, many people find that the side effects of pain-relieving drugs are often too high a price to pay. For years, researchers have been looking for a way to deal with pain without side effects. Currently, pain relief is one of the hottest areas of medical research—because there is a huge need for analgesia and because when this huge need is met, the result is profit. Pharmaceutical companies as well as manufacturers of other kinds of remedies, such as magnets and electromagnetic devices, see an especially profitable future in supplying pain relief medications as the baby boomers get older.

The biggest generation in human history is about to enter late middle age. This group is already encountering the grim reality of the aging process and its effects on muscle, tendon, and bone. This reality is only going to get worse for millions of people. Mix the inevitability of aging with the expectation of this generation for living a full, active, sexy, and fun life, and you have a recipe for a huge need for pain relievers. Baby boomers want to play golf until they are ninety, and they don't want to get a stomach ulcer in the process by taking too many pain-relieving drugs. Could magnets be the answer?

There is now a wealth of anecdotal evidence supporting the usefulness of magnets in helping with pain relief. Many high-profile athletes, golfers in particular, have publicly discussed their use of magnets for sports injuries and long-term wear and tear, popularizing the idea that magnets are effective.

The worldwide market for magnets is expanding rapidly—individuals in North America alone spent $200 million on magnets in 1998. Worldwide sales are estimated at around $5 billion. Yet, until recently, there was very little scientific evidence to support the use of magnets for pain relief, and, until recently, no research had been undertaken at a reputable American medical institution.

Then in 1997, a study on magnets and pain was published in the *Journal of the American Academy of Physical Medicine and Rehabilitation*.[1] The study, which was conducted at the Baylor College of Medicine in Houston, Texas, by Drs. Carlos Vallbona, Carlton Hazlewood, and Gabor Jurida, provoked considerable interest among America's physicians.

THE BAYLOR MAGNET STUDY

The Baylor Magnet Study appears to offer proof that magnets can relieve pain. The study made doctors and researchers sit up and take notice. Was there really something to this ridiculous idea of using magnets? Was magnet therapy, after all, a bona fide way of treating pain? Before the study, it would be fair to say that the vast majority of doctors thought permanent magnets were yet another form of quackery designed to liberate dollars from the pockets of gullible citizens. The Baylor Study made them think otherwise.

Carlton Hazlewood has a Ph.D. in physiology and is an organism physiologist. In an interview I conducted with him, he said, "[Being an organism physiologist] means I know the whole body; I didn't just specialize in one area. I evolved into a molecular physiologist and biophysicist, but I always have been primarily interested in the whole organism, and that's why I got into magnets."

Hazlewood has long been a proponent of the new view of the living cell, a controversial theory that is too complex to go into here, but that has marked him as somewhat of a maverick in the scientific community: "I have grown to learn that whenever the scientific community comes out and beats its chest and says something ain't possible, it usually is." For several years, Hazlewood, one of the developers of the MRI, had been curious about the medical use of magnetism. In the early 1990s, he was on the NIH/NOACM committee for investigating electromagnetism, and he served on the panel for bioelectromagnetic applications in medicine. He also had a personal interest in investigating the pain-relieving properties of magnets:

> I have enormous patella [knee] pain. I was a steel storage tank builder, that's how I worked my way through undergraduate college, and then I paid my way through graduate school as a professional wrestler, which I did for three years. I spent most of my young life abusing my body tremendously and, as a result, suffer from chronic pain now.
>
> Sometime in 1993, I found out about trigger points, and I found that there was one in the groin that referred to the patella. I taped a magnet onto this trigger point as an experiment, and within 20 minutes I had no pain in my knee. This was stag-gering to me. So I wanted to create a study that would test two hypotheses: that magnets relieve pain and that magnets placed on the trigger points relieve specific pain.

Dr. Hazlewood was joined in this study by Carlos Vallbona, a pediatric cardiologist and a colleague of Hazlewood's at the Baylor College of Medicine in Houston, Texas. Vallbona had also had severe knee pain and at one point could hardly walk. Hazlewood told me that he placed a couple of magnets on Vallbona, who was then able to walk within minutes.

The Baylor Study was notable for two of its criteria. First, a notable restriction on the study was that the response to the magnets had to occur within 45 minutes. The second criterion was that the magnets had to be placed on trigger points, which are areas in muscle that cause pain elsewhere when pressed. Sometimes trigger points are on or very close to a pain site, and sometimes they are in another area, such as the groin trigger point that Hazlewood used to treat his knee pain. Seventy percent of trigger points correlate with acupuncture points.[2,3]

Vallbona and Hazlewood were aware of previous studies that had been performed using electromagnetic fields in various orthopedic conditions. One of these studies was the 1938 Hansen study, in which 23 of 26 patients with complaints of sciatica, lumbago, and arthralgia reported significant pain relief from the use of magnets. This study was only a single-blind, meaning that the two patients who did not get the electromagnetic treatment didn't know, but the doctor did. But all the same, these two patients reported no pain reduction, in stark difference to those who did receive the treatment.[4]

In the treatment of osteoarthritis, double-blind, placebo-controlled studies (using the PST system, see chapter 9) have shown that a pulsed electromagnetic field can relieve pain.[5,6]

With these studies to encourage them, in addition to their subjective experience of using magnets for their own pain, Hazlewood and Vallbona set about devising a study on magnets that would meet modern standards of scientific method.

How the Baylor Study Was Conducted

All fifty patients who took part in the study had been diagnosed with post-polio syndrome, meaning that at one time in their lives they had suffered from the infectious disease poliomyelitis, which had left them with chronic muscular or arthritic-like pain. Either an active (really a magnet) or a placebo (a device that just looked like a magnet) was applied to a pain site for 45 minutes.

This study was a double-blind pilot study and a randomized clinical trial, which means it met the standards of the modern scientific method. *Pilot* means that the study wasn't a very big one. In fact, the study used only 50 patients. *Randomized* means that determining who got the magnets and who did not was completely random. *Clinical* means the study took place in a clinic. *Double-blind* means that neither the doctors nor the patients knew if what was being used was a real or a fake magnet.

Of the patients, 29 received real magnets, and 21 received fake ones. The BIOflex magnet company provided the doctors with magnets that had codes on the back.[7] Only by reading the code could someone determine whether it was a real magnet, and that code was not broken until all patients had completed their part of the study. Of course, anyone with a paper clip could have held the clip to the "magnet" to see if it was real. Therefore, Vallbona and his research associates insisted that patients were watched and that any sneaky testing did not occur.

What Is Post-Polio Syndrome?

People with post-polio syndrome frequently suffer from pain in the joints due to degenerative arthritis caused by age and by the long-standing, asymmetrical load on the joints caused by polio. The most common type of joint pain occurs in the lower back, the neck, and the sacroiliac joint. People with this condition also often have hip and shoulder pain. They may also experience muscular pain, which can be evaluated by palpation of the reported sore muscles and by identifying specific trigger points associated with the referred pain. The results of the Baylor Study are relevant to anyone who suffers from any kind of muscular or joint pain, regardless of the cause.

The Magnets Used in the Study

The magnets supplied by the BIOflex magnet company had a pattern of concentrically arranged circles of alternating polarity. The company gave the study team 8 discs, 40mm in diameter and 1.5mm thick; 18 discs, 90mm in diameter and 1.5mm thick; 20 credit-card–sized pads, 83mm by 53mm and 1.5mm thick; and 24 strips, 175mm by 50mm and 1.5mm thick.

The 40mm discs and the strips had a magnetic field intensity of 500 gauss each. The 90mm discs and the credit-card pads were rated as 300 gauss. There were an equal number of placebo devices that were identical in size and shape to the active magnets. Each device, whether real or fake, was placed in a number-coded envelope and delivered to the researchers in four separate boxes, according to the shape of the magnet. The code numbers that identified which devices were active magnets and which were inactive were not broken until the study was completed.

The Participants in the Study

To be eligible for the experiment, patients had to have had significant pain for at least four weeks immediately prior to the study. They had to have a fairly normal body weight—less than 140 percent of the normal weight for their age and height. (This requirement was made because it is thought that if there is a great deal of fat between the magnet and the site of pain, then the magnet won't work as well.) The patients could not take an analgesic or similar drug for at least three hours before the study.

How Pain Was Measured

Each patient chose one pain site to which the device was applied, even though the patients often had multiple areas of pain. When patients reported pain in more than one area, the area most sensitive to touch was selected. Patients were not given any explanation about what the expected response might be, but they were told that their level of pain at that site would be tested by palpation of a trigger point before and after the device was applied.

The researchers located an active trigger point associated with the site of referred pain by prodding with a finger and by firmly applying a blunt object approximately one centimeter in diameter. Prodding in nonpainful areas would produce a sensation of pressure but no pain.

Each subject was asked to grade the pain subjectively at the trigger point, using the McGill Pain Questionnaire, which employs a scale from 1 to 10 (with 1 being the least painful and 10 being the most).

Performing the Study

Once the pain site and trigger point had been determined, the doctors applied the appropriate-sized device—a disc, a credit-card–sized pad, or a strip-shaped device. An envelope containing a device of the appropriate shape was randomly selected from a box and applied to the skin with adhesive tape.

The subjects stayed in the clinic or immediate area and were told to keep the device in place for the next 45 minutes. They were instructed to assume any position or action that was most comfortable, including walking. After 45 minutes, the device was removed, and the subjects were asked to report whatever sensations were felt while the device was on them. Then the trigger points were pressed again, and the patients were asked to gauge the intensity of the pain. The same McGill scale of 1 to 10 was used. At all times, the investigators tried to be as consistent as possible in the amount of pressure they applied to the trigger points.

Results of the Baylor Study

Patients who received active magnets reported an average pain score decrease of 4.4, plus or minus 3.1, on the 10-point scale. Those with the placebo devices experienced a reduction in pain of 1.1, plus or minus 1.6, on the 10-point scale. This is a substantial difference between the two groups, and, assuming that the study was done properly, it is a difference that cannot be explained by the placebo effect. The proportion of patients in the active-device group who reported a pain-score decrease greater than the average placebo effect was 76 percent, compared with 19 percent in the placebo-device group.

The researchers concluded, "The application of a device delivering static magnetic fields of 300 to 500 gauss over a pain trigger point results in significant and prompt relief of pain in post-polio subjects. Whether the pain was of a myofascial or arthritic nature, it seemed to respond equally well to the static magnetic field, and the effect was noticed within 45 minutes from the onset of the application."[8]

In addition, patients who had more than one area of pain often reported relief in other areas, even though there was no magnet there. This was especially true with people who had sacroiliac pain on both sides and who had the magnet applied to the side that was most sore. Those people felt relief on the other side as well. Although this is a very interesting finding, Vallbona hesitates to make much of it, saying that the matter needs more research. According to Vallbona, quoted in an interview published in *Arthritis Today,* "There's no question in my mind that magnets hold great promise."

He agreed that more studies are required and stressed that the Baylor Study was just the beginning.

Conclusions Drawn by the Baylor Study

The Baylor Study report concluded:

> The delivery of static magnetic fields through a magnetized device directly applied to a pain-trigger point or to a localized painful area results in significant relief of pain within a short period of time (less than 45 minutes in our study) and with no apparent side effects. Based on the results of this study and reports in the literature of the effect on people with arthritis, it appears that magnetic field energy may be useful in the management of pain in individuals with other types of impairments that are commonly treated in primary care settings.[9]

According to Vallbona:

> The majority of patients in the study who received treatment with a magnet reported a significant decrease in pain, and most of the patients who were given a placebo, or inactive magnet, reported very little or no improvement. . . .
>
> We don't have a clear explanation for the significant and quick pain relief observed by the patients in our study. . . . It's possible that the magnetic energy affects the pain receptors in the joints or muscles or lowers the sensation of pain in the brain.[10]

Possible Problems with the Baylor Study

Some critics have said that the previous experience of Vallbona and Hazlewood with magnets on their own injuries may have corrupted their objectivity.[11] According to the critics, Vallbona and Hazlewood were predisposed to finding that magnets work for relieving pain. As was discussed in chapter 4, it is well documented that the bias of the researcher has an effect on the outcome of an experiment. Although this factor, in itself, does not nullify the results of the Baylor Study, it does mean that, operating within the rules of modern scientific method, the study should be replicated before the results are taken to be foolproof.

It is important to point out, however, that with a new form of therapy like magnets (at least, new to conventional Western medicine), unless the researchers have had positive experiences themselves, it is less likely that the research would be initiated in the first place.

An additional factor is the difficulty of achieving objectivity in pain studies. Any study of pain is inherently difficult to assess, given the subjective nature of the experience of pain itself.

The Future of Research on Magnets and Pain Relief

The Baylor research team has suggested several areas that need more research. The team would like to see the following issues addressed directly:

1. What is the relationship between strength of magnet and length of time of application for pain relief?
2. How long does the positive effect last?
3. What are the local and central effects of magnetic fields on the same pain area?
4. What is the effect of the simultaneous application of magnets on several pain-trigger areas?

5. Do the size and shape of a magnetized device alter its effectiveness?

6. What is the cost-effectiveness of managing pain using magnetic fields versus traditional pharmacological or physical therapy modalities?

SUMMARY

Researchers have been working for years to come up with a pain-relieving drug with minimal side effects and long-lasting effectiveness. The Baylor Study suggests that it is the humble magnet that has the power to provide us with the remedy we have all been looking for.

6

Magnets and Fibromyalgia
The Colbert Study

Fibromyalgia is a painful condition that affects the whole body. The main symptoms are muscular and bone pain, stiffness of the joints, disturbed sleep, and fatigue. Millions of people are afflicted by this debilitating condition. In the United States, 3.4 percent of women and 2 percent of the population as a whole suffer from the disease.[1] The cause of the disease is not known, and it is notoriously difficult to treat. Once the disease has developed, many sufferers never fully recover.

There have been anecdotal reports that magnetic mattress pads both enhance sleep and diminish pain, and so, logically enough, many people with fibromyalgia have been drawn to try them. People using magnets began to report that they were experiencing benefits, so researchers have become curious about the usefulness of this treatment.

If you have looked at Web sites that sell magnetic products, you may have come across an abstract of a study by a Dr. Kazuo Shimodaira (an abstract is a brief synopsis of a research study). Shimodaira's abstract describes a twelve-month, double-blind study of 431 patients that was reportedly undertaken in Tokyo in 1990.

Although Dr. Shimodaira does not mention fibromyalgia specifically, all the patients in the study suffered from fatigue, insomnia, and chronic pain. In the study, 375 patients were given real magnetic pads, and 56 were given nonmagnetic pads. The study showed that after a patient slept on a magnetic mattress pad for three days, there was a noticeable reduction in pain in 80 percent of cases and improvement in sleep in 64 percent of cases. The patients continued using the pads for twelve months, and apparently the beneficial effects continued to be felt, with no side effects.

Dr. Shimodaira's study has been widely reported on the Internet, and most sellers of magnetic mattress pads include the abstract on their Web sites. I wanted to make sure the abstract was authentic, and I also wanted to read the full study, so I wrote to Dr. Shimodaira in Japan. The mail was returned as undeliverable. So I contacted a colleague in Tokyo and asked her to try to track down the doctor. Despite repeated attempts, she was unable to find him. Officials at the hospitals mentioned in the study said they didn't know of him. This doesn't mean the study is not authentic. A great deal can happen in ten years. All I know for sure is that Dr. Shimodaira is hard to find today, and without the full report, it is not possible to judge how reliable the study really is. However, whether or not it is a valid study, it has provoked a good deal of interest among sufferers of fibromyalgia and among their doctors.

A more recent study at the University of Virginia, by Ann Gill Taylor, R.N., funded by the National Institutes for Health (NIH), concluded that there were no clear findings to support the use of magnetic mattress pads. The study was presented at the November 1999 Vanderbilt Conference on Magnet Therapy. Researchers present at the conference told me that they found the presentation of the study to be unconvincing and that it appeared to have been poorly designed.

As of January 2000, the Gill study had not yet found a publisher, which suggests that it may be too flawed to merit inclusion in a peer-reviewed journal.

Given that many medical journals are only too happy to publish negative studies about magnets and that the research has not been refunded, one can only conclude that there was a problem with the design and/or the actual performance of the study. Taylor did not return my calls, so I wasn't able to obtain any information about the study from her directly.

Another study, by Dr. Agatha Colbert of Tufts University School of Medicine in Boston, was published in the *Journal of Back and Musculoskeletal Rehabilitation* in February 2000. This chapter closely examines the Colbert Study for what it can tell us about fibromyalgia and magnets.

THE COLBERT STUDY ON FIBROMYALGIA

Agatha Colbert, M.D., is clinical assistant professor of physical medicine and rehabilitation at Tufts University School of Medicine, Boston. In 1997, she ran a pilot study using magnetic mattress pads to treat the pain and sleeplessness of fibromyalgia. This study is important and noteworthy because it was well-constructed. It was thorough and met all of the research criteria mentioned in chapter 4—repeatable, placebo-controlled, double-blind, and randomized. The study also gives clear evidence that magnets can help this difficult and debilitating condition.

As well as being a medical doctor and a teaching professor, Colbert is also an acupuncturist in private practice in Waltham, Massachusetts. She first became interested in acupuncture when she was working in the chronic pain program at Spaulding Rehabilitation Hospital. In an interview I had with Dr. Colbert, she mentioned, "I felt there had to be something else that would help people with chronic pain." Her studies in acupuncture led her to investigate magnets. She has been using magnets for about five years, treating about 300 patients along the way.

Her experiences with using magnets were sufficiently positive that she decided to set up a clinical trial using magnetic mattress pads. "My background is in rehabilitation, so I'm very interested in therapies that people can use at home." As Colbert notes in the study, "Pharmaceutical management strategies for treating patients with fibromyalgia have limited success and a high incidence of associated adverse effects," which gives good reason to explore alternative methods.[2]

In performing the study, Dr. Colbert was assisted and advised by Marko Markov, Ph.D. (Department of Orthopedics, Mount Sinai School of Medicine, New York); Mandira Banerji, M.A. (research assistant, Litterst & Associates, Newton, MA); and Arthur Pilla, Ph.D. (Department of Orthopedics, Mount Sinai School of Medicine, New York; Department of Biomedical Engineering, Columbia University, New York).

The primary objective of the study was to find out if the chronic pain and sleep disturbances experienced by people with fibromyalgia improve when they sleep on magnetic mattress pads. Every night for 16 weeks, subjects slept at their homes on a special mattress pad. The experimental group slept on real magnetic pads; the control group, on sham (nonmagnetized) pads.

Design and Approval

The Colbert Study was a double-blind, placebo-controlled, and randomized pilot study. The study was approved by the Tufts University School of Medicine Investigational Review Board through the Department of Physical Medicine and Rehabilitation.

The Subjects

The 35 initial subjects were all women with fibromyalgia. They were recruited from three sources: Dr. Colbert's clinical practice, a referring physical therapy group, and a local fibromyalgia support group. Thirty of the women met the criteria and were accepted for participation in the study. Out of this group, 25 completed the study. Five had to drop out: one withdrew on her own, one was withdrawn because of a psychiatric hospitalization that happened during the study, and three others were disqualified because they broke rules of the study. The average age of the 25 subjects who completed the study was 49.7 years (the youngest was 25 and the eldest was 78). The average weight was 166 pounds, with a range from 115 to 216 pounds. All the subjects had had chronic and widespread pain symptoms for at least 2 years.

Inclusion/Exclusion Criteria

To qualify for the study, the subjects had to meet the diagnostic criteria for fibromyalgia syndrome designated by the American College of Rheumatology.[3] This meant that they had to have had pain for longer than 3 months, and pain had to be present on both the right and left sides of the body and both above and below the waist.

In addition, the subjects had to agree to start no new pain medications or additional pain management treatments during the 16-week trial period. They were allowed to continue with current medications or therapies, such as physical therapy, acupuncture, chiropractic, or myofascial release, but only if they had started them at least 4 weeks before the study began.

How the Study Was Performed

This study was performed at the patient's homes and at Dr. Colbert's private practice. The subjects were randomly assigned to either the experimental or the control group.

The mattress pads—either genuine or sham—were shipped directly to the subjects' homes. The experimental and the sham mattress pads looked exactly the same. The codes identifying which mattresses were real and which were sham were kept by the manufacturer until all the data had been entered into the computer system. Once the information was in the system, the data were sent to a biostatistician who had no contact with the subjects.

Neither Dr. Colbert nor her research assistant, Mandira Banerji, came in contact with any of the mattress pads. They both remained blinded observers throughout the clinical assessments and data analysis phases, meaning they did not know which subjects had the real pads and which did not. During the entire course of the study, neither the subjects nor the researchers had any contact with the manufacturer or the biostatistician.

At the start of the study, Dr. Colbert gave all the women an initial clinical examination to confirm the diagnosis of fibromyalgia. They were also seen for two follow-up visits: after 2 weeks of sleeping on the mattress and again for a final evaluation at the end of the 4-month trial period.

Each of the women in the study slept on the pad every night for 16 weeks. The women were told to use the mattress pad only at night and not to rest on it during the day. Every week, the subjects mailed in the results for that week, filling out charts to describe their general well-being, incidence of pain, sleep disturbance, fatigue, and tiredness on waking. Most of the subjects kept in weekly phone communication with Dr. Colbert and Banerji. The patients were told not to talk about the study if they happened to meet another participant.

The Mattress Pads

Both the experimental and sham mattress pads were provided by Magnetherapy, Inc. Each pad contained

270 domino-shaped, ceramic pieces, measuring 2.0 by 4.5 by 1 cm. The ceramic pieces were placed 4 cm apart and were arranged in a pattern of 15 columns and 18 rows. All of the ceramic pieces were encased in the bottom layer of two layers of hospital-grade foam, which were glued together. The entire pad was covered by a quilted cotton case. The total thickness of the mattress pad was 4 cm.

The ceramic pieces in the mattress pads of the experimental group were magnetized with a surface-field strength of 1100 ± 50 gauss each. With this surface-field strength and the positioning of magnets in the pad, Colbert and her colleagues estimated that between 200 and 600 gauss were actually delivered to the skin surface from each magnet. As Colbert notes in her report, "This magnetic field level is well within that reported to achieve clinically meaningful therapeutic effects." To support this assertion, Colbert cites the Baylor Study, mentioned in chapter 5, and the Weintraub study, described in chapter 8.[4,5]

The magnets in the pad were placed in such a way that the field direction facing the body repelled a north-seeking compass needle. This is the direction usually identified as north among magnet users, but called a south polar direction traditionally. Some clinicians have found that this "north" direction has a calming, soothing, and pain-relieving effect on tissue. The sham pads contained the same number and same shape of ceramic pieces, but the pieces were not magnetized.

Dr. Colbert asked all the subjects in the study to resist trying to determine whether they had a real pad. She instructed each subject to place the pad on the bed in the position indicated on the label as soon as it was delivered directly from the manufacturer. If placed properly, the thickest foam layer of the pad was on top, making it difficult to detect magnetization with lightweight items, such as paper clips. Therefore, any casual occurrence, such as a metal object falling on the pad and being magnetized, would not happen.

Evaluating Pain and Sleep Changes

The study used four methods to measure the responses of the subjects in the study: Visual Analog Scales (VAS), Total Myalgic Score, Pain Distribution Drawings, and a modified Fibromyalgia Impact Questionnaire (FIQ). Visual Analog Scales are a standard method used by doctors to assess the various factors involved in fibromyalgia. The scales consist of a series of different diagrams for five factors: global well-being, pain, sleep, fatigue, and tiredness upon waking. The subjects had to place a mark at the point on the scale for each topic to represent their symptom level for that day.

Because people with fibromyalgia often experience a wide fluctuation in day-to-day symptoms, the subjects were told to complete the VAS on Wednesdays at about 10:00 A.M. Most people with chronic ailments experience swings in symptoms over the weekend because of family factors, change in routine, and so forth, so the subjects were specifically requested not to record the VAS on the weekend. The completed VAS was mailed every week to Dr. Colbert's office, where the results were entered into a database.

In addition to the subjective VAS reports, tests were done that had some objective value. The Total Myalgic Score method of evaluating pain in fibromyalgia measures pain at 18 specified tender points. The examiner uses 4 kilograms of digital pressure to determine if the point is sore when pressed. (The digital pressure of 4 kilograms is the point at which the thumbnail begins to go white.) For a confirmed diagnosis of fibromyalgia, there must be 11 out of 18 points that are painful. Colbert did this test on the subjects when she met them at the beginning of the study. The intensity of tender-point pain was scored as 2 for intense pain, 1 for moderate pain, and 0 for no pain at these points. The total possible myalgic score was 36 if all the tested tender points were described as intensely painful. These total myalgic scores were retested at the end of the study.

The third method, Pain Distribution Drawing, employs color to access a different level of awareness than the more straightforward Visual Analog scales. The subjects had to color in a line drawing of a body from the front, back, and side views. They used red to indicate severe pain, green to indicate moderate pain, and no color where there was no pain. Colbert and Banerji created a template that they superimposed on the drawings in order to quantify the pain shown by the coloring. The template consisted of 316 contiguous circles. The researchers then counted the number of colored circles for a total score. Red circles were scored as 2 and green circles as 1. One coloring was done at the start of the trial, and another at the end.

The fourth, and final, method of evaluating symptoms was the Fibromyalgia Impact Questionnaire, a physical functioning test. This test was developed by Burckhardt, Clark, and Bennett in order to assess the current health status of people with fibromyalgia.[6] Dr. Colbert used the first part of this questionnaire, employing ten questions to assess physical functioning in tasks of daily living. The best possible score is 0, meaning subjects are always able to do the ten specified tasks of daily living. The worst possible score is 30, meaning they are never able to perform any of the tasks. All the subjects completed the modified FIQ at the beginning and end of the trial period. Dr. Colbert also asked the subjects to keep a daily diary and to record any unusual or adverse reactions.

Results

When the results were all analyzed, it became clear that the thirteen subjects who had been sleeping on the experimental mattress pads had experienced a significant decrease in both pain and fatigue. They showed significant improvement in sleep and in performing tasks of daily living. The twelve subjects who had been sleeping on the sham mattress pads experienced no significant change in the same areas.

By the fourth week, subjects in the experimental group showed a significant reduction in pain. Their pain continued to lessen through week 12, with no further improvement by week 16 (the end of the trial). Overall, they experienced a pain reduction of 32 percent. In contrast, the control group using the sham mattress pads experienced no significant change in pain throughout the entire 16-week period.

In terms of sleep, the experimental group was showing a significant improvement by week 12, with a further improvement by week 16, to give an overall figure of a 40 percent improvement. The control group showed no improvement in sleep.

The experimental group showed improvement in fatigue by week 8, and this state was maintained, with no further improvement, up to week 16. Fatigue lessened on average by 42 percent. Once again, the control group showed no difference.

Interestingly, both groups showed improvement in tiredness on waking: 39 percent in the experimental group and 21 percent in the control group. This suggests that tiredness on waking is a symptom that is highly influenced by state of mind. There was clearly a placebo effect operating in this particular parameter of the study. This particular placebo effect has been reported in other clinical trials on fibromyalgia.[7,8,9]

Also interesting—given the claims by some magnet proponents that magnets improve general well-being—

neither group experienced any effect on global well-being. This is curious: one would think that getting more sleep and being in less pain would help you feel better overall.

Side Effects

When Colbert reviewed the daily diaries and spoke with the subjects, she found that there had been no apparent adverse effects due to the magnetic mattress pad. Three of the participants, all of whom had received the active pads, found that their usual symptoms intensified for a period. For the first seven to ten days, they had an increased incidence of aches, pains, and fatigue. The symptoms then subsided, and the subjects felt increasingly better. A number of people have reported a similar experience. Some believe this phenomenon indicates a detoxifying effect provoked by the magnets stimulating the circulation of lymph, blood, or both. According to Dr. Colbert:

> This type of "therapeutic exacerbation," a phenomenon observed by osteopathic physicians, chiropractors, physical therapists, and other body workers, is characterized by a temporary worsening of symptoms during the initial weeks of treatment. We are postulating that the small perturbations in the body's bioelectromagnetic field caused by magnet placement may be evoking the same type of self-limited "therapeutic exacerbation." The two recruits who initially excluded themselves from the study had previously experienced an exacerbation of symptoms while using permanent magnets on certain acupuncture points. They reported increased pain, nausea, and dizziness while wearing the magnets but obtained almost immediate relief of the symptoms when the magnets were removed. There are other reports of certain individuals who are particularly sensitive

to electromagnetic fields. This appears to be a sub-set of the population who should be identified and studied further.[11]

Conclusions

The researchers concluded: "Sleeping on a magnetic mattress pad, with a magnet surface field strength of 1100 ± 50 gauss, delivering 200–600 gauss at the skin surface, provides statistically significant and clinically relevant pain relief and sleep improvement in subjects with fibromyalgia. No adverse reactions were noted during the 16-week trial period."[10]

HOW DO MAGNETIC MATTRESS PADS COMPARE WITH DRUG THERAPIES?

The results of Colbert's study are particularly notable when compared with drug trials on fibromyalgia. Rates of improvement with drug trials are quite low, occurring in only 25 percent of subjects taking tricyclic medications and other central nervous system active medications.[12] In addition, these medications become less effective over time. Side effects are experienced by as many as 98 percent of patients.[13]

OTHER FACTORS TO CONSIDER WHEN WEIGHING THE COLBERT STUDY

The researchers had to factor in the possible effect of the firm mattress pad itself. Indeed, subjects in both groups reported enjoying increased comfort from the hardness of the mattress pad for the first half of the study period. This correlated with improvement in fatigue on the VAS in both groups. However, this effect leveled off by week 8 in the control group, while the experimental group continued to improve over the entire 16-week trial, showing that there was an effect on fatigue from the magnets, not simply from the firmness of the pad.

Dr. Colbert and her colleagues discussed the limitations of their study in their report and made recommendations for future studies.

> The limitations in this exploratory study suggest recommendations for future studies. Stricter selection criteria should be implemented to exclude: subjects who are on morphine-like drugs; subjects who are involved in significant life changes such as marriage or divorce; anyone in the process of settling a medical disability claim; and subjects in whom a psychiatric disorder is a dominant feature.
>
> A certain range of weight should also be a selection criterion in order to assure minimal baseline differences between the groups. Subjects should have baseline VAS scores of at least 4 so as to eliminate a floor effect, i.e., when patient entry scores show low levels of impairment or discomfort, there is little room for measurable improvement. In addition, a lead-in assessment time for the two-week period prior to actually using the mattress pads would provide a more reliable baseline. Actual duration of time spent on the mattress pads and usual sleeping position should be more precisely documented.[14]

FURTHER RESEARCH

The Colbert research team recommended that follow-up trials be undertaken.

> Because pharmaceutical agents are associated with a high rate of adverse effects and offer only minimum relief for the majority of patients, we

recommend a trial of magnet therapy, as a noninvasive, painless, low-risk adjunct to standard medical and psychiatric interventions.

Further controlled investigation of devices, which incorporate permanent magnets for the treatment of chronic and acute musculoskeletal pain, is definitely warranted. A minimum study period of 2 years is recommended to document long-term efficacy, assess the possibility for habituation, and determine optimal dosimetry, including strength of magnetic fields, exposure time, and pole orientation. In this manner, the efficacy of this promising, simple, noninvasive treatment for FM may be properly established.[15]

SUMMARY

We've looked at this study in depth and have seen how it gives some significant hope for the management of fibromyalgia symptoms. Chapter 7 examines more studies that show how magnets can help in other conditions and situations, including diabetic neuropathy, the healing of wounds, and postoperative bruising and inflammation.

7

Magnets and Wound Healing
The Man Study

For several decades, electrical and magnetic fields have been used to assist the healing of bone, but the role of magnets in healing soft tissue has not been investigated until recently. If it were found that magnets could have a similar effect on soft tissue as they do on bone—speeding and enabling the healing of problematic wounds—it would mark a revolutionary breakthrough in several areas of medicine.

Wound healing is a major issue in plastic surgery. It can sometimes take several weeks, even months, for tissue to heal completely, and until that happens the patient suffers from unsightly bruising, swelling, and accompanying pain and discomfort.

Dr. Daniel Man is a board-certified plastic surgeon who has been in practice in Boca Raton, Florida, since 1981. In recent years he has been investigating the use of permanent magnets to help with healing of tissue after surgery.

Originally from Israel, Dr. Man is an innovative and dedicated surgeon who is also an artist of some note. (One of his paintings hangs in the White House.) In addition to his pioneering work with magnets, he has also developed a new face-lift technique (called the Man face-lift expander) that avoids stretching of the mouth. He has also invented an implantable homing device, which uses the global satellite system, for use on humans.

Like Carlton Hazlewood and Carlos Vallbona, Dr. Man first became interested in using magnets because of a personal experience. Curious about how magnets might work for his patients, he asked someone who knew about magnets to come to his house. At that time, Man's wife had an injured knee from an automobile accident and was suffering from a great deal of pain, which nothing seemed to help. They decided to experiment on her knee with a magnet and were amazed to find that the pain went away within two minutes. Impressed by this result, Man decided to set up a small trial to test how magnets could help with wound healing after surgery. He suspected that a similar electrical mechanism might operate in soft tissue healing as is known to occur in bone injuries.

Man's initial pilot study was not double-blind nor was there a control group. The subjects were 21 of his patients who had just received various cosmetic plastic surgical procedures, including face-lifts and liposuction.

Man and his colleagues, Harvey Plosker, M.D., and Boris Man, M.D., used magnets that delivered 150 to 400 gauss to the target tissue. The magnets were arranged within soft pads, which were placed on each patient over the area that had been operated on.[1]

In eight cases, the patches were applied before pain was felt, and in thirteen cases the patches were placed on the area after pain, swelling, and/or bruising had begun to appear. The patches were attached with light dressings and left for 48 hours. The treated area was inspected at 24, 36, 48, and 72 hours following the operation.

The results of this pilot study were promising. In about 60 percent of the patients, there was a reduction in pain, swelling, and bruising, and in 75 percent of patients, pain and swelling disappeared completely. Patients needed fewer painkillers than is usual after these types of surgery. Where there was severe bruising, the application of the magnets appeared to speed healing considerably. Encouraged by these results, Dr. Man set up a further study.

THE MAN STUDY

Design and Approval

The Man Study was double-blind, placebo-controlled, and randomized. The Essex Institutional Review Board approved the protocol for the study. There were twenty patients in the study, each of whom had undergone suction lipectomy (commonly known as liposuction). The major complications of liposuction are postoperative pain, swelling, and bruising.

Exclusion/Inclusion Criteria

To be included, patients had to be between 18 and 75 years old. They were excluded if they were unable to give informed consent or if they had a pacemaker, open wounds, infection, major medical problems, metallic implants at the treatment site, and/or skeletal immaturity.

How the Study Was Performed

All the patients in the study received liposuction surgery from the same doctor, using a two-to-one ratio of tumescent solution and ultrasound. Areas treated included the abdomen, saddlebags, love handles, and thighs. There were two groups of ten patients each in the study. The patients were randomly assigned to a group. One group had active magnetic patches placed over the site of the surgery, and the second group had inactive, sham devices placed in exactly the same way.

The control devices looked and felt identical to the active devices.

The patches varied in size from 5 by 15 cm to 20 by 30 cm and were the same strength and style of patches as were used in the pilot study. The patches contained ceramic magnets with a north (or negative) polarity on the side that was placed on the skin. Immediately after surgery, the patches were placed over the area that had been suctioned and were left in place for fourteen days.

Evaluating the Results

The treated areas were inspected on days 1, 2, 3, 4, 7, and 14. At each inspection, pain, edema (swelling), and ecchymosis (discoloration) were evaluated. The same observer, who had no idea which devices were real and which were sham, made all the postoperative assessments. All the participants were blinded—that is, neither the patients nor the observer nor the surgeon knew which magnetic pads were active.

Discoloration was measured on a scale of 0 to 10, with 0 representing a normal skin appearance and 10 representing severe discoloration with no normal skin color showing through.

Swelling was measured by comparing the operated area with nearby tissue, again on a scale of 0 to 10. A measurement of 0 represented no edema compared with surrounding tissue, and 10 represented a high level of swelling, with the skin looking shiny due to being stretched by the fluid in the tissues.

Pain was measured by a visual analog pain scale. (See chapter 6 for a description of VAS.)

Results

When the study was completed and the blind broken, the researchers found that the two study groups were similar in terms of age, gender, and extent of the liposuction performed. In the treatment group—the group that received the active magnetic devices—there was a statistically significant reduction in discoloration when compared with the control group on postoperative days 1, 2, and 3. By postoperative days 4, 7, and 14, there was no longer any significant difference in discoloration between the two groups.

Similarly, there was a statistically significant reduction in edema (swelling) on days 1, 2, 3, and 4. By days 7 and 14, there continued to be further reduction in edema, but it was no longer statistically meaningful.

With the pain measurement, the researchers found that pain was significantly decreased on days 1, 2, 3, 4, and 7. The patients in the treatment group also took notably fewer painkillers. There was no difference in the incidence of complications in both groups, and no side effects were observed in either group.[2]

The results of the study were quite stunning. The healing process was significantly accelerated. The patients who received the active magnet devices experienced healing of their postoperative bruising and swelling in two to three days, rather than the usual two to three weeks. In addition, they had to take far fewer pain medications.

Implementing the Findings

Dr. Man told me that following this successful research, he now uses this method of magnet therapy on all liposuction and face-lift patients.

> We are working under the theory that when there has been an injury or damage to an area, which of course includes surgery, the body generates an electrical current that stimulates healing. By adding a magnetic field to this naturally occurring current, it appears that the healing is accelerated.

The swelling goes down faster, and the patients feel less pain. The magnet operates as a feedback mechanism, which causes the natural healing process to get going faster.

Often after plastic surgery, there can be considerable pain, and this method helps us make the procedure better for patients and cuts down on the medication they need. This in turn helps the body normalize faster.

It seems that by some mechanism the magnets improve the blood supply to the area, which results in a reduction in swelling, which in turn causes a reduction in pain. The magnetism has an anti-inflammatory effect and increases the amount of oxygen that gets into the tissues.

So far, Dr. Man has had a mixed reaction from his peers. The journal that published his study, the *Journal of Plastic and Reconstructive Surgery,* is the most prestigious publication in the field, so there is clearly major interest in his work. But while most doctors are not outwardly skeptical, many are still cautious. One colleague reported Man to the ethics committee of the AMA following a television interview in which Man had said that magnets appeared to be a useful and low-cost way of speeding postoperative healing. Following a peer review, Man was completely exonerated. Coincidentally, one of the members of the investigating committee revealed that he himself had had a powerful experience using a magnet on a difficult-to-heal wound that was a complication of diabetes.

Dr. Man is currently engaged in developing further research into the use of magnets in other types of plastic and reconstructive surgery. "So far, I have found that the face responds very nicely, and that many areas that have been suctioned respond very well." His immediate next step is to do further research in methodology to find out what strength and shape of magnets work best on what body parts. Dr. Man's pioneering work has great implications for other types of surgery and medical conditions, as well as for healing after accidents.

8

More Scientific
Evidence on Static Magnets

Arthur Pilla is a biophysicist on the faculty of Columbia University. He was involved in very early investigations into the use of pulsed electromagnetic fields and bone repair. He has been doing extensive research into electromagnetism and health for nearly thirty years. Dr. Pilla gave me a useful overview of the current magnet research scene. He began by talking about his own experiences in the lab with static magnetic fields:

> I think it's all real at this point, very much so; but I didn't start off that way. I used to be very skeptical about the usefulness of static magnetic fields, but in recent years I've seen results in my own lab.
>
> Around eight years ago, we started some research and by accident, very much by accident actually, discovered that very weak magnetic fields had a significant effect on an enzyme system that we were studying. We pursued it and dug in quite deeply. This is what persuaded me that it is worth investigating static magnets and the clinical applications.

I spoke with several other scientists and physicians and gathered the most convincing evidence from recent research into static magnets. I've already discussed at length the Baylor Study into magnets and pain, the

Colbert Study into magnets and fibromyalgia, and Daniel Man's studies into wound healing after plastic surgery. This chapter describes more briefly some other credible studies into the medical uses of static magnets.

One study, which has provoked considerable interest, was performed by Dr. Michael Weintraub in 1998.

MAGNETS AND PERIPHERAL NEUROPATHY

Dr. Michael Weintraub's 1998 study on the use of magnets for diabetic peripheral neuropathy was published in the *American Journal of Pain Management*.[1] His study showed promising results using magnetic foot insoles to treat nerve damage in people with diabetes.

What Is Peripheral Neuropathy?

Peripheral neuropathy is a complaint that affects millions of people. It is a painful nerve condition that often affects the extremities, especially the feet, but that can ultimately affect every nerve in the body. It causes burning, tingling, prickling, numbness, and even sharp, jabbing pains. In some cases it causes loss of balance, muscle weakness, difficulty walking, and extreme sensitivity to touch. These problems result from damage to the peripheral nerves of the body, which are the long, fragile nerves that extend out from the spinal cord and connect the whole body to the central nervous system.

Peripheral nerves can be damaged by many factors, including certain illnesses, as well as the side effects of medication, exposure to toxic substances, and alcoholism. Peripheral neuropathy is a common complication of diabetes. Other vulnerable groups include people who are HIV positive, those who have AIDS, those with rheumatoid arthritis, and people who suffer from a host of other autoimmune disorders.

Peripheral neuropathy is difficult to treat. Conventional treatment is often ineffective and includes the use of antidepressants, analgesics (both narcotic and non-narcotic), anticonvulsants, and acupuncture. Most of these treatments have never been clinically tested. A 1998 study at the Terry Beirn Community Programs for Clinical Research on AIDS found that neither amitriptyline (a commonly used treatment for the problem) nor acupuncture, nor a combination of the two, proved to be effective.

Weintraub's Study

Weintraub's study was a randomized, double-blind, placebo-controlled, crossover study. (In this instance, *crossover* refers to a part of the study in which the subjects had an active magnetic insole for one foot and an inactive one for the other. After a predetermined time, the insoles were switched. See below for more details.) The study was designed to test the effectiveness of magnet therapy in relieving the pain of peripheral neuropathy and also to assess the role of placebo.

Of 24 initial patients, 19 completed the four-month trial. There were 10 patients with diabetic peripheral neuropathy (DPN) and 9 patients with non-DPN (i.e., peripheral neuropathy due to a cause other than diabetes, such as those described above). All the subjects had tried other remedies for their neuropathy, without experiencing any improvement. All of them had failed to get better using conventional pharmacological treatments, and a few had also tried acupuncture, to no avail.

The subjects were randomly given an active magnetic foot insole (with a manufacturer rating of 475 gauss) for one foot and a similar-appearing sham insole for the other foot. The subjects scored their incidence of burning, numbness, and tingling pain independently in each foot twice a day. After thirty days, the insoles were switched for another four weeks. At the end of the second month, subjects returned the first pair of insoles and were given a new set consisting of two active insoles (475 gauss each) and continued for eight weeks, rating their levels of pain and discomfort twice daily. During this four-month period, no new therapeutic interventions, such as new drugs, were permitted.

In addition to the subjects making their own assessment of their conditions, they were examined and assessed once a month by Dr. Weintraub. Nerve testing was also carried out to see if objective criteria matched the reports of the subjects.

The study used Magstep brand magnetic foot insoles, manufactured by Nikken. These insoles are 475 gauss in strength and consist of alternating poles arranged in a geometric triangular design. The insoles have a penetration depth of $1^3/4$ inches (4 cm). Weintraub was working on the theory that magnets in this type of insole induce a current that stimulates both blood vessels and nerves. (Although as far as physicists are concerned, static magnetic fields do not induce a current, as explained in chapter 3.)

Subjects were instructed to wear the insoles as close to the soles of their feet as possible, twenty-four hours a day, seven days a week, for four months.

Results

Interestingly, the diabetics in the study improved more than the other subjects, and by a significant margin. This result suggests that peripheral neuropathy caused by diabetes is particularly responsive to magnet therapy. Of the 10 diabetic subjects, 9 (90 percent) experienced statistically significant reductions and/or resolutions of their symptoms of burning pain, numbness, and tingling. Of the 9 nondiabetic subjects, 33 percent showed equivalent improvement. In a previous non–placebo-controlled study that he conducted, Weintraub found that out of 14 subjects overall, 75 percent of the diabetic group and 50 percent of the nondiabetic group experienced significant relief.

MAGNETS AND THE SIDE EFFECTS OF CHEMOTHERAPY: A CHINESE STUDY

A study conducted in China and reported in the *Journal of Traditional Chinese Medicine* in 1991 showed that magnets help alleviate the side effects of chemotherapy.[2] In the study, researchers placed magnetic disks on the point known as Neiguan, or Pericardium 6 (P6), the most often-used acupuncture point for nausea and vomiting. This point is situated about 2 inches up the inside of the arm from the center of the wrist. Neiguan is known to many Westerners, as well as to just about everyone in China, Korea, and Japan, because of the anti–travel-sickness aids that have been marketed during the past decade. These aids are taped to the inside of the arm and stimulate Neiguan.

All the patients in the study were taking cisplatin, a commonly used chemotherapy drug that often causes side effects, chiefly, nausea and vomiting. Antinausea drugs can hinder the chemotherapy from working properly, so there is no completely satisfactory conventional treatment for this debilitating side effect. The researchers tried several methods to alleviate this problem, and it was when they tried magnets on Neiguan that they found a solution. They found that the treatment had "a remarkable effect."

All the subjects in the study had moderately advanced or advanced cancer, treated by 20 mg of cisplatin daily for five days, followed by an interval of three to four weeks between sessions. Most patients received three bouts of the chemotherapy, thereby taking three months to complete the entire course of treatment. Patients who experienced nausea and vomiting were given 20 to 40 mg of paspartin (an antinausea drug) intramuscularly. Those who received no benefit from paspartin were chosen to take part in the study and were divided into three groups. The first group received magnet therapy; the second, fake magnet therapy; and the third, point compression (acupressure) over Neiguan, the same point that in the first group was being stimulated by the magnet.

The first group had 161 patients; the second group, 23; and the third group, 22. Of the 161 patients in the magnet therapy group, 53 were male and 108 were female, ranging in age from 11 to 82 years and averaging 52.7 years. Of the 45 cases comprising the other two groups combined, 11 were male and 34 female, ranging in age from 11 to 75 years, averaging 55.8 years. Types of cancer were found proportionately in each group.

Method of Treatment

For the magnet therapy group, a flat magnet was sewn to a cotton band. The magnet was a disk 5 mm thick and 20 mm in diameter that measured 600 gauss in strength. The magnet was placed on the arm that was not receiving the chemotherapy drip, with the north pole of the magnet facing directly onto the skin, exactly on the Neiguan point. The band was tied onto the arm just before the patient began receiving cisplatin via the drip and was removed two hours after all the chemotherapy had been administered. Usually the band was in place for six to eight hours. It was fastened just tightly enough to avoid any effect on blood circulation.

For the nonmagnet group, a similar cotton band with a disk of the identical size but made of ordinary iron was attached in the same manner. In the compression group, a steel ball with a diameter of 0.5 cm was used instead of a disk. The three types of bands were applied in the same way for the same length of time.

Results of Treatment

Treatment was considered to be *very effective* when there was no longer any experience of nausea or vomiting following cisplatin intake, *effective* when nausea and vomiting were mild, and *ineffective* when the nausea and vomiting were just as bad as before. Of the 161 cases in the magnet therapy group, the treatment was very effective in 99 cases (61.4 percent), effective in 45 (28 percent), and ineffective in 17 (10.6 percent). Of the 23 cases in the nonmagnet group (the placebo group), the therapy was very effective in no cases at all, effective in 5 cases (21.7 percent), and ineffective in the remaining 17 cases. Of the 22 cases in the point compression group, none received any relief. In the magnet therapy group, no side effects were observed.

This study showed the results of using a magnet on Neiguan to be 89.4 percent effective, which is far higher than any drug currently available or than any other kind of therapy known so far. The fact that pressure had no effect, when it is known to have an effect in milder forms of nausea, shows how difficult it is to treat nausea induced by cisplatin.

As noted by the writers of the research paper, "The method is effective, safe, and painless. It can even be manipulated by the patient himself and is widely applicable in clinical practice."[3]

MAGNETS AND WOUND HEALING: A CASE STUDY OF A GUNSHOT WOUND

Dr. Richard Rogachefsky of the Department of Orthopedic Surgery at the Jackson Memorial Hospital at the University of Miami, Florida, performed this case study. Rogachefsky's patient was a seventy-year-old man with a gunshot wound to the left hand. The man had a severe fracture in his left hand and a large, open wound. The surgeon operated to remove all dead soft tissue and bone, and the patient was put onto a drip of antibiotics. x-ray showed that most of the first metacarpal bone was destroyed, making the joint between the thumb and first finger completely unstable.

A week later the surgeon performed a bone graft from the patient's pelvis to the injured hand to stabilize the thumb and to give the patient the use of his hand. On the fourth day after this surgery, Dr. Rogachefsky placed a permanent magnet (Tectonic brand) over the region of the thumb of the bone graft and over the open wound. The magnet was left in place for the duration of the treatment. After five weeks, the bone graft had completely integrated with the existing structures, and the wound had completely healed.

Usually in a wound of this magnitude, fusion would take at least two to three months. This wound healed extremely quickly, in merely one month. Dr. Rogachefsky attributed the result to the effect of the magnetic field stimulation on the bone graft.

When I asked Dr. Rogachefsky how he thought this result may have occurred, he said, "I don't know how magnets work, but I'm seeing really good results with them. In the case of the gunshot wound, magnets definitely accelerated the healing of both the fracture and the wound by at least ten days."[4] Rogachefsky is in the process of completing two clinical trials using magnets on wound healing, the results of which will be available in the spring of 2000.

MAGNETS AND MENSTRUAL PAIN

A study at South Korean University, performed in 1992 and published in a peer-reviewed Korean medical journal, showed promising results for the treatment of menstrual pain.[5] The investigator, Dr. Kim Lee, designed a small placebo-controlled study that took place over five months. The subjects were assigned randomly to one of two groups. Group 1 consisted of 11 women who were each given an active magnet of 800 to 1,299 gauss. The control group had a sham magnet. The pain levels of both groups were assessed using three different pain-rating scales.

At 9:00 A.M. on the morning following the onset of menstrual pain, the subjects came to the doctor's office to have their pain level measured. Then they put the devices on the area just above the pubic bone, on the lumbar area of the lower back, and on a point four inches above the inner ankle. Pain was measured three hours later, at which point the magnets were removed. Pain was again measured another three hours after the magnets had been taken off.

The results showed a significant difference in the pain scores between the treatment group and the placebo group at both three-hour measuring times.

MAGNETS AND PREMATURE BABIES: A CASE STUDY

Diane Cody and James Moran conducted an interesting case study in 1998 in Massachusetts. The study was published in the *Neonatal Network* journal.[6] Diane

Cody is a registered staff nurse at the Baystate Medical Center in Springfield, Massachusetts. James Moran is an acupuncturist at the Baystate Medical Center who has been working with static magnets for the past fifteen years. (Read more on his work in chapter 12.)

Cody and Moran teamed up to see if magnets could help Baby Alex, born May 30, 1998, after only 26 weeks in utero. At the request of Alex's parents, magnets were used on him daily, beginning when he was 72 days old.

Shortly after birth, Alex developed severe bronchopulmonary dyspasia (BPD) and was put on ventilation support. He received standard medical care for the BPD, and after 12 weeks magnet therapy was introduced. Alex slept on a 14-by-24-inch pad that had 40 flat rectangular magnets inside. Each magnet had strength rated at 3,950 gauss, but probably measured between 600 and 1,000 gauss at the surface. All the magnets had the north pole facing Alex and the south pole facing the bed. In addition, a large 4-by-6-inch magnet, half an inch wide, was placed on the bed 3 inches above Alex's head so that the north pole of the magnet faced him. This large magnet also had a manufacturer's rating of 3,950 gauss but, again, was most probably between 600 and 1,000 gauss at the surface.

Two main findings were noted. First, Alex's muscle tone became much more relaxed. Before the magnets were applied, Alex had very tight shoulder and neck muscles and was sensitive to any touch. This is common in BPD infants, who often have such pronounced muscle tension their backs arch. After the magnets were applied, Alex's caregivers found that he became much more relaxed and was able to be handled comfortably.

Second, Alex grew rapidly. One of the effects of BPD is that it slows growth considerably. The slope of Alex's growth curve got steeper after the magnet therapy began. Moran thinks that there may be a magnetic effect that stimulates secretion of human growth hormone: "This may, in part, account for Alex's increased growth rate."

Alex died of unknown causes at 125 days. Despite his death, the study is considered a success because of his progress up to that point. The fatality rate among such tiny premature newborns is tremendously high, and no one considers his death to have anything to do with the magnet therapy. The success of this one case has been sufficient to draw in funding for a full-scale, double-blind, placebo-controlled study to begin in 2000.

SUMMARY

These studies, though small, present a picture of magnets as a serious therapeutic tool under certain circumstances. To clearly identify those circumstances, we need to examine the field of pulsed-electromagnetic therapy, in which far more research has been undertaken.

9

Pulsing Electromagnetic Field Therapy

There is a growing amount of data on magnetic field therapy using pulsing electromagnetic fields (PEMFs) on certain parts of the body. Although this book focuses on the use of permanent (or static) magnets, research on pulsing magnetic fields is also of interest to the degree that it shows that magnetic fields do have a substantial impact on the human organism. In addition, at least one of the devices currently being developed, the Enermed device, is designed for use by the consumer.

We know more about PEMFs simply because more people have studied them, more money has been available, and more research has been done. Pulsing electromagnetic fields are more complex than simple magnetic fields. With a PEMF, the magnetic field is not static; rather, it is time-varying. This enables the magnetic field to induce electrical fields and currents. Each aspect of the PEMF, as well as the combination of the magnetic and electrical fields with the accompanying electrical current, may have a beneficial effect on the body. PEMF technology was first developed to heal bone fractures and has since been employed for other orthopedic conditions and for soft tissue repair.

Over the past two decades, much attention has focused on the potential health effects of electromagnetic fields. There has been considerable consumer concern, press coverage, and scientific research about the electromagnetic fields created by power lines, mobile phones, microwaves, computers, and other appliances. We still don't know to what extent such electromagnetic waves may be harmful. At this point, the evidence suggests that the effects, if any, are minimal.

Research on electromagnetic fields has been contradictory and influenced by the vested concerns of business corporations and by the desire of the consumer for greater convenience and comfort in daily life. This is a big topic that I won't go into here, other than to say that research is ongoing and still inconclusive. What we do know about electromagnetic fields is that at this time we have far more evidence of the healing effects than of any harmful ones. As far as the healing aspect goes, researchers and physicians are gradually beginning to understand and harness this useful therapeutic tool.

In Russia and eastern Europe, research into electromagnetic fields (EMFs) has been ongoing since World War II: "In Russia, a vastly different political, economic, and social situation resulted paradoxically in giving their scientists far more democratic and academic freedom (and funding) than their Western counterparts in choosing the focus of their research efforts, without interference from vested interests."[1]

In the United States, research into EMFs—pulsing or otherwise—did not get going until the 1960s, when it was discovered that injured bone creates tiny electrical currents as it heals. As a result of this discovery, most of the research associated with EMFs and the human body has focused around bone fractures, osteoporosis, and osteoarthritis. Recent EMF studies have extended into brain research, with several studies examining how EMFs can help depression, epilepsy, and schizophrenia. Some studies suggest that EMFs may also help multiple sclerosis and migraines.

The studies described in this chapter tell us something about the usefulness of pulsing electromagnetic fields, but as with permanent magnets, the amount of research is not yet conclusive. However, the research does provide a solid indication of a highly promising therapy. More research needs to be done before we will know both the extent of the therapeutic benefit and any possible side effects.

BONE-RELATED DISORDERS

Nonunion Fractures

In the early 1970s, Robert Becker, Andrew Bassett, and Carl Brighton successfully demonstrated that electrical stimulus (direct current) helps nonunion bone fractures to heal. *Nonunion* means that the bone has failed to heal, and such fractures are notoriously difficult to treat.

Later that decade, Andrew Bassett and Arthur Pilla developed the use of pulsing electromagnetic fields to heal bone. With this technique, the electromagnetic field can be delivered without electrodes touching the body. Instead, a field is generated from a coiled wire placed near the body. Bassett and Pilla experimented with a wide variety of electromagnetic fields and found four frequencies that stimulate fractures to heal. They chose the frequency that worked best for their therapeutic device, which was approved by the FDA in 1979.

The method developed by Bassett and Pilla uses alternating current supplied in bursts of pulses to direct the electromagnetic field. At the same time as this technique was accepted, the FDA also approved the use of direct electrical current. According to Robert Becker, both methods work equally well, although the PEMF method using the coil is simpler for the patient to use. In any event, the use of electromagnetic fields to heal nonunion fractures is now a standard treatment.[2, 3]

Osteoarthritis

A 1993 study by Kenneth Miner and Richard Markoll, reported in the *Journal of Rheumatology,* showed promising results in the use of pulsed electromagnetic fields on people with osteoarthritis (OA). The researchers noted that, for more than a decade, magnetic fields have been used as a treatment for delayed-union fractures, and so the fields might be useful for healing the worn-down bone that occurs in OA.

In this pilot, double-blind, randomized trial, 27 patients with OA, primarily of the knee, were treated with PEMF. Treatment consisted of eighteen 30-minute periods of exposure that took place for approximately one month, using the Pulsed Signal Therapy (PST) device, a specially designed, noncontact, air-coil device. Observations were made on six clinical variables at the beginning of treatment, halfway through, at the end, and one month later. Twenty-five patients completed the treatment.

The results were quite impressive. The patients who received treatment from the active device showed an improvement in the clinical variables ranging from 23 to 61 percent. The patients who were given the nonactive, sham device experienced an improvement of 2 to 18 percent. No toxicity was observed.

The researchers concluded: "The decreased pain and improved functional performance of treated patients suggest that this configuration of PEMF has potential as an effective method of improving symptoms in patients with OA. This method warrants further clinical investigation."[4]

A further double-blind study completed by David Trock, Alfred Bollet, and Richard Markoll in 1994 confirmed these initial findings, and the PST has been in use in Europe ever since. The manufacturer is awaiting FDA approval in order to be able to use the device in the United States.[5]

Osteoporosis

In the late 1990s, a year-long study took place at the Creighton University School of Medicine in Omaha, Nebraska. In the study, 52 subjects spent 20 minutes a day on a vibrating platform, which is thought to stimulate bone growth by triggering the production of tiny electrical fields within the bone. The study showed promising results for the use of PEMF for treating osteoporosis. Other studies on sheep and rats indicate that electromagnetic field therapy is a potentially important breakthrough in the treatment of osteoporosis.[6]

BRAIN-RELATED DISORDERS

Several studies have been conducted using transcranial magnetic stimulation (TMS), a technique that uses an electromagnetic copper coil device to stimulate the brain. The device is placed on the scalp over the desired area, and an electrical current is passed through the wire coil. This technique has the effect of generating a pulsed magnetic field that induces electric currents in the brain, causing changes in the targeted areas.

The field of transcranial magnetic stimulation is growing rapidly, and researchers are examining its potential usefulness in several areas of neuropsychiatry. There are centers conducting studies into TMS in Australia, Israel, Switzerland, Germany, the United

States, and the United Kingdom. Current research is examining the use of TMS in treating depression, epilepsy, Parkinson's disease, schizophrenia, and post-traumatic stress and obsessive-compulsive disorders. All of this research is also helping us to understand the complex nature of the frontal part of the brain—the prefrontal cortex, the area in which so many of our mental functions take place.

Depression

Neurologists have found that many people who suffer from depression have less activity in the frontal cortex of the brain, relative to people who are not depressed. Several studies over the past few years have demonstrated that electromagnetic stimulation to the affected part of the brain can have a beneficial effect upon depression.

Dr. Pascual-Leone, an associate professor at Harvard Medical School and a researcher at Beth Israel Deaconness Hospital, undertook a study in 1996 attempting to show how TMS can help with severe depression. The subjects in the trial were people on whom drug therapy had been ineffective. Pascual-Leone and his colleagues used repetitive transcranial magnetic stimulation (rTMS). So far, the results have been promising. Pascual-Leone found that a 10-day course of treatment had long-term effects. Half of his patients felt an improvement that lasted for three to four months.[7]

An Israeli study published in 1999 in the *Archives of General Psychiatry* also showed that this treatment is effective for depression. The Israeli study was a double-blind, placebo-controlled study in which 70 subjects with major depression were assigned to either rTMS or sham treatments of 10 daily five-minute sessions over two weeks. The rTMS group was given stimulation on the right prefrontal cortex at a frequency of 1 hertz, with 0.1-millisecond pulse duration. Sixty-seven subjects completed the experiment. Of the 35 in the rTMS group, 17 (49 percent) experienced at least a 50 percent improvement in their depression. Only 8 out of the 32 in the sham group experienced a similar benefit.[8]

These studies have been conducted on patients with severe depression. No one knows if this technique is useful for people with mild depression.

TMS has been well-tolerated by patients, with none of the risks associated with electroconvulsive therapy. The beneficial effects of TMS usually last three to four months after each course of treatment.

Epilepsy

A 1999 study undertaken in Gottingen, Germany, showed that pulsed magnetic stimulus applied to the top of the head reduced seizures in people with severe epilepsy. Epilepsy is caused by excessive activity in one part of the brain, which overloads the brain's circuitry leading to seizure—in effect, a short circuit. The study was very small, involving only nine participants. Nonetheless, the results were so striking that they caused immediate interest in the medical community.

Severe epilepsy is life-threatening and can be very difficult to treat. Each of the nine participants in the study had such a severe case of epilepsy that it could not be completely controlled with medication. On average, each participant had seven seizures per week in the six months prior to the study.

The researchers investigated the use of rTMS, which induces lasting effects on cortical excitability, meaning that it calms down the brain. The researchers thought it possible that rTMS might reduce seizures, as epilepsy is associated with extreme excitability of the brain. It seems they were right.

Of the nine participants, five were women, and four were men. They were aged 21 to 48 years old. For four weeks before and after the treatment, the participants recorded every definite seizure or seizure-like event. For the purposes of the study, every partial seizure was counted as a seizure. During the period of the study, medication was kept constant.

The rTMS was administered once a day for five consecutive days. Each day, two trains of 500 pulses from a repetitive magnetic stimulator were applied via a round coil 9 cm in diameter onto the top (vertex) of the head.

None of the nine participants suffered any adverse reaction to the rTMS therapy. Out of the nine, eight reported a drop in number and severity of seizures. Two patients showed no reduction in numbers of attacks. One patient showed a decrease of 20 percent, two showed a decrease of 20 to 50 percent, and three patients experienced a reduction of the weekly seizure rate of more than 50 percent. This change was short-term, and by six to eight weeks after the rTMS had been applied, all the participants had returned to their pre-study seizure levels.

The researchers concluded that "low-frequency rTMS may temporarily improve intractable epilepsy." They are currently engaged in placebo-controlled studies to confirm these initial findings. Low-frequency magnetism was used because high frequencies are suspected of triggering epileptic seizures.

Although the study was simply a pilot study, it is still important on two counts. One, the results were dramatic, suggesting that magnetic fields do have a very real effect on brain function. Two, the success of the study meant that larger, double-blind, clinical studies would get funding.

It is estimated that up to a quarter of all epileptics cannot control their fits through medication. This breakthrough concept of using pulsing magnetic field therapy could have a hugely beneficial effect on the lives of this population.[9]

Schizophrenia

A study published in the *Lancet* in March 2000 reported promising results treating schizophrenia with TMS. The study, performed by Ralph Hoffman and colleagues at Yale University, focused on auditory hallucinations, a commonly found symptom among schizophrenics that causes distress and inability to control behavior. About 50 to 70 percent of schizophrenics report auditory hallucinations, often in the form of hearing voices, which sometimes "tell" the sufferer to perform destructive acts upon themselves and others.

Twelve patients who had daily auditory hallucinations received 1-hertz transcranial magnetic stimulation to the left temporoparietal cortex—the area of the brain known to be active during auditory hallucinations. The researchers used a low-frequency magnetic field, and the treatment was applied for 4 minutes the first day, increasing daily until, by the fourth day, they were receiving the treatment for 16 minutes a day. As a control, two to three days after completing the active course of treatment, the same patients went through a sham course for the same length of time.

There was a significant difference in results between the active and the sham treatments. Patients reported a notable improvement after receiving 12 to 16 minutes of TMS but noticed no benefit from the simulated treatment. All but one patient experienced a reduction of the severity of the hallucinations. In eight patients, the hallucinations ceased entirely for a period of time ranging from four days to two months.

Hoffman and his team continue to research this promising therapy. They are investigating whether auditory hallucinations can be controlled over longer periods of time and whether TMS can help with other symptoms of schizophrenia.[10]

MULTIPLE SCLEROSIS

A 1997 study by Dr. Todd Richards, Dr. Martha Lappin, and associates at the University of Washington showed promising results for the treatment of some of the symptoms associated with multiple sclerosis. This double-blind study involved 30 patients, half of whom were given an inactive device. The Enermed brand device used in the study delivers a pulsing magnetic field with a very low frequency (4–13 hertz), delivering a 50–100 milligauss peak magnetic field. The device is a small (1.62 by 1.75 by 0.5 inches), battery-operated, pulsed magnetic field generator.

The results of the study showed a significant improvement in the treatment group versus the control group for the following symptoms: bladder control, cognitive function, fatigue level, mobility, spasticity, and vision. There was also a significant change pre- and post-treatment in alpha EEG magnitude during the language task recorded at various electrode sites on the left side.[11]

MIGRAINES

The Enermed device is also being used to treat migraines with some success. Dr. Martha Lappin, one of the researchers on the multiple sclerosis study, did a study on migraine sufferers in England in 1994–1995. The study was performed via survey questionnaire, a method that is difficult to assess for two main reasons: (1) the report by the patient is entirely subjective, and (2) patients who fail to reply to the questionnaire may be the ones who failed to find any benefit. People are more likely to answer a questionnaire if they have something significant to report. In this study, no objective findings were measured, and there was no control group, so the placebo effect may be significant.

Despite these drawbacks, the survey results indicate that the Enermed device was useful. Almost two-thirds of the respondents reported substantial improvement after they started using the device. The positive results were most striking among those who suffered from severe migraines.

ELECTROMAGNETIC DEVICES

Apart from those devices used in bone repair, all the other electromagnetic field devices detailed in this chapter are only available in clinical trials in the United States, while the manufacturers and the medical profession await FDA approval. Currently, all the other electromagnetic devices mentioned in this book are only available in other countries.

The Enermed device, used in the studies on multiple sclerosis and migraines, was developed in Britain and is available there and in Canada.

The Pulsed Signal Therapy machine, invented by Dr. Richard Markoll, is widely used outside the United States and is designed for use by trained medical personnel. Magnetherapy, Inc., the manufacturer of the PST, claims that the device has been used on 75,000 people in 250 clinics in Europe. Magnetherapy says the device has also been used on many horses.

The Jacobson Resonator Unit is also available in Europe. Designed for use by physicians, this device was in the news in 1998 when Mohammed Ali, suffering from Parkinson's disease, abruptly ended a course of treatment using the device, claiming that the company was using him for publicity. The inventor, Dr. Jerry Jacobson, claims that the device regenerates certain genes that shut down after childhood, regenerating the patient's brain cells and causing them to produce dopamine. (Parkinson's disease is caused by a lack of dopamine.[12]) Dr. Jacobson claims to have patents on his devices in 80 countries and says he is engaged in ongoing research at many universities and colleges of medicine. He and his colleagues are doing research into regeneration of myelin sheath in nerves (currently by studying mice), and they have also recently completed a double-blind study on epilepsy in Oklahoma, for which a positive result is anticipated. The Oklahoma study was a pilot study with about a dozen people. Unlike other researchers, Jacobson works with extremely low frequencies of electromagnetism.

The companies that have developed these magnetic pulsing devices and that are awaiting FDA approval are hopeful that the approval will come through by 2001. It looks likely that simple devices for the consumer will be available in the not-too-distant future, along with more complex devices designed for use by physicians and surgeons.

The field of electromagnetic therapy has much to offer the health-care consumer. As Dr. Arthur Pilla pointed out when I interviewed him, "Using electromagnetic fields for bone repair costs ten to twenty times less than a bone graft and has an equal chance of success as the first bone graft. It is noninvasive, nonoperative, and take-home. I'm very proud of my part on the development of this technique. . . . If we can continue in that vein, we'll be doing very well." Pilla envisions a future in which disposable bandages are devised that incorporate a tiny electromagnetic field device. These bandages would be available from pharmacies and would be used for all kinds of problems, ranging from ankle sprains to bedsores.

As well as the potential for speeding the healing of injuries, simple electromagnetic therapy devices for other problems, such as migraines and osteoarthritis, may also soon become available for the consumer. Many of the other conditions detailed in this chapter would be amenable to home treatment once the right devices have been developed and approved.

SUMMARY

As we can see from all the studies described here, electromagnetic therapies are applicable for several disorders and diseases that, until now, have proved difficult or impossible to treat. This is an exciting development in medical care. As research continues, we can expect to see an increase in the use of this therapy for a wider range of conditions.

Part 3

Practical Applications

10

When to Use Magnets

This chapter covers several issues concerning the use of magnets. First, we'll look at the issue of self-care and the question of whether you should use magnets by yourself or with the advice of a health-care professional. Second, we'll look at which types of conditions have shown themselves to be amenable to treatment from magnet therapy. Third, there is a section on the contraindications for using magnets, detailing information about when you should not use them. Finally, we'll examine what is currently known about safety and side effects.

SELF-CARE AND MAGNETS

I am very much in favor of informed self-care in medicine. In many cases, people can use magnetic devices to treat themselves successfully for minor ailments. However, for any long-term or serious health problem, you should seek consultation with a medical professional. Even if a complaint is relatively minor, there are significant advantages to using magnets with the advice of a doctor of either traditional or alternative medicine. A professional who has studied magnets will be able to determine the most effective kind of magnetic device for your condition and will be able to monitor the effects of the magnets. For example, an acupuncturist can put magnets on you and then read your pulses (a Chinese diagnostic technique) twenty or thirty minutes later and detect if the magnets have had a beneficial effect and to what extent. Likewise, a chiropractor can check the range of movement, gauge the level of inflammation, or use applied kinesiology before and after the magnet is applied.

Medical professionals who are experienced with using magnets can also determine if you are one of the rare people for whom magnets act as an irritant. For some people, use of magnets may actually be harmful. A study by Stanislav Schmigelsky, published in Poland in the mid-1980s, found that a small proportion of the population (0.002 percent) has an adverse reaction to magnetic fields. This is the result from only one study, however, and future studies along these lines may reveal a higher or lower incidence of sensitivity, especially among certain sectors of the population.

Dr. Agatha Colbert, chief investigator of the fibromyalgia study discussed in chapter 6, has used magnets on more than 300 patients. She has found that there is a small proportion of people who are highly sensitive to magnetic fields. Such people experience magnets as irritating and overstimulating. These people may find that they only need to use the magnets for a very short time for there to be a beneficial effect. Others have found that magnets are ineffective but leave them feeling a bit jangled. In the latter case, the patients usually settled back down after a few minutes. (The safety and side effects of magnets are discussed in more detail at the end of this chapter.)

Magnet therapy is a rapidly growing field, but many doctors may not have kept up with the latest research. In some parts of the United States, there may not be any medical professionals with thorough knowledge of magnets, in which case you have no choice but to go it alone. In light of Dr. Colbert's comments regarding sensitivity, if you are going to use magnets on your own, it's important to monitor yourself carefully. If you feel that the magnet has been on long enough, take it off. If the magnet makes the pain worse, take it off. If it feels irritating, take it off. You may wish to reapply the magnets later and see what happens. We all have different tolerances for different kinds of medication and therapy. Most people seem to derive only benefits from magnet therapy, and many doctors and scientists seem convinced that there are no deleterious side effects. But that doesn't mean you should ignore your own instincts and feelings.

If you are going it alone, this book will help you keep a level-headed approach to magnets. The information in this chapter will help build your confidence about using magnets by yourself.

WHEN TO USE MAGNETS

Scientific research tells us that applying magnets can help relieve pain; reduce inflammation and swelling; accelerate the healing of scar tissue, bruises, and broken bones; and stimulate circulation in certain disorders. Anecdotal evidence indicates that magnets may help an even wider range of conditions. In this book alone, there are case studies showing that magnets have provided relief or aided complete resolution of bedsores, cellulite formation, old scarring, lack of mental clarity, sense of physical weakness, and other conditions.

Although some people and some sources claim that magnets can help every disease and disorder known to humankind, studies and anecdotal evidence suggest this is not so. As with any system of medicine, magnets are effective for certain conditions and ineffective for others. Magnets may be useful for more conditions than are mentioned in this book, but the following list details situations in which they have frequently proven helpful.

- Arthritis
- Back pain: acute and chronic
- Neck and shoulder pain: acute and chronic
- Knee pain: acute and chronic
- Bone injuries: fractures, bruising of the bone
- Soft tissue injuries: tendinitis, sprains, bruises
- Insomnia
- Fatigue
- Menstrual pain
- Fibromyalgia
- Scar tissue
- Edema: swelling, water retention
- Post-surgical wound healing
- Conditions involving inflammation

WHEN MAGNETS ARE NOT A GOOD IDEA: CONTRAINDICATIONS

There are three instances in which magnets should not be used.

1. *If you are pregnant.* This preclusion is made out of caution due to the lack of total and certain proof that magnets can be used safely during pregnancy. Although there is nothing to suggest they cannot, ever since the Thalidomide disaster, the medical community has been very cautious about recommending any treatment unless it has been thoroughly proven to be safe in pregnancy. Even though one study showed that magnetic fields could affect DNA in mammalian cell cultures, all other studies, and many have been done, have shown the reverse to be true; that is, static magnetic fields do not cause DNA changes or genotoxicity.[1,2] To date, there is no proof

that static magnets affect human DNA in live tissue. Similarly, there is no evidence that magnets might be deleterious to the pregnancy, the mother, or the baby. But still, we should continue to err on the side of caution, and so doctors recommend that pregnant women should not use magnet therapy.

2. *If you have a pacemaker or other kind of electronic implanted device, such as an insulin pump.* This is a definite contraindication. The electronics in pacemakers and other devices can be upset by the magnetic field emanating from the magnet.

3. *If you have epileptic seizures.* Some people with epilepsy may be extra sensitive to magnetic energy, so caution is recommended. We do not really know whether magnets are dangerous for people with epilepsy. The most recent research suggests that low-level doses of magnetic energy (as is delivered through a static magnet) may actually be good for people with epilepsy. Low-level pulsating electromagnetic fields have been shown to reduce the number of seizures in people with severe epilepsy. But until the evidence is clearer, caution is advisable.

ARE MAGNETS SAFE?

The vast majority of research scientists and medical practitioners today hold that static magnets are safe when used at therapeutic strengths (up to 20,000 gauss). There has been extensive research into this subject during the past two decades. One stimulus for research has been the need to make sure that MRI machines, which emit very high levels of magnetism, are safe for both patients and clinicians.

Dr. John E. Moulder, professor of radiation oncology at the Medical College of Wisconsin, has made an exhaustive review of the many studies done on static magnetic fields. He concludes that at therapeutic dosages, static magnetic fields are safe.[3]

The World Health Organization reported, "The available evidence indicates the absence of any adverse effects on human health due to exposure to static magnetic fields up to 2 tesla [20,000 gauss]."[4]

Carlos Vallbona and his colleagues at the Baylor College of Medicine concluded in their study on magnets and post-polio syndrome:

> The fact that none of our patients reported any discomfort resulting from the use of magnetic devices and that no complications have been reported in the literature supports the notion that low-intensity magnetic fields produced by permanent magnets or electromagnetic devices are biologically safe.[5]

For this book, I interviewed several scientists and researchers about what they thought about magnet safety. I found that there was a wide range of opinions.

Arthur Pilla, a pioneering researcher into magnets and magnetism, thinks there is no reason to fear magnets: "All of these signals, including the signals we use for bone repair, are all very weak, in the scheme of things. Even the power line controversy is not really turning out to be very much, and I'm glad, because the therapeutic benefits of all these fields far outweigh any of the risks that anyone can imagine."

Richard Hammerschlag, who holds a Ph.D. in biochemistry, gave me a much more cautious answer. Hammerschlag is a prominent researcher in the field of complementary and alternative medicine. He is research director at the Oregon College of Oriental Medicine and president of the Society for Acupuncture Research. On the subject of therapeutic magnets, he said, "We're just beginning to understand the subtle energies of the body. To go and blithely slap magnets on yourself without any research on side effects seems a little premature and possibly risky."

The Bulgarian physicist, Dr. Marko Markov, has been doing research into the therapeutic properties of magnetic fields for more than thirty years. When describing the Polish study on sensitivity, mentioned earlier in this chapter, he told me, "This kind of result [from the Schmigelsky study] is another reason why I don't want magnets to be in the hands of businesspeople; I want it to be in the hands of the medical community. As with any therapeutic modality, the therapist needs to control what happens with the patient." Markov has concerns about people buying magnets in stores and using them without medical advice: "Using magnets without understanding the therapeutic nature of the magnetic fields is inadvisable."

Markov's perspective arises not because he thinks magnets are dangerous but because he thinks the efficacy of the treatment is compromised by lack of knowledge. In fact, he thinks that use of magnets is a very safe form of therapy: "Medicine applied to the outside of the body, such as magnets and acupuncture, even if it does have a systemic effect on the body, is much safer than a pill, which goes into the bloodstream and is immediately systemic."

Markov is convinced that an overdose of a magnetic field is not possible: "If you give the body a magnetic field that it does not need, the body will ignore it." In addition, he maintains that overdoses aren't based on duration of use because the body adjusts to the magnetic field. In fact, the magnetic field stops having a therapeutic effect. It stops being a stimulus. "In order to be a stimulus, [the magnetic field] needs to come and go."

On the other end of the safety spectrum is the radical view on the dangers of magnets held by Jerry Jacobson, D.D.S. and inventor of the Jacobson Resonator Unit (discussed in chapter 9). Jacobson claims that his very low-amplitude electromagnetic method is safer than any other technique because it mimics the normal electromagnetic fields of the body. He holds a strong and highly controversial opinion about safety. In a phone interview, he told me, "The amplitude of the magnetic field in conjunction with the frequency can create a window through which carcinogenesis can occur."

Jacobson thinks that static magnets are potentially cancer-forming and believes that they are too strong for the body, even at a low rating of 300 gauss. I include Jacobson's viewpoint to give a full picture of the kind of thinking present today among magnet researchers. It must be said, however, that there is no convincing research to back up his assertions. And, as he owns the patent on the one device that, in his opinion, is safe, his objectivity is called into question. On the other hand, his questioning of the consensus view is a good thing in that it acts as a spur to prove more thoroughly that static magnets are as safe as people think they are.

John Upledger, a well-known osteopath and teacher of the Upledger method of craniosacral manipulation, holds a somewhat more measured, but still cautious, view. Upledger argues, "Long-term use of external magnets can cause autonomic systems to change their set points. When the magnetic fields are removed, the set points require significant time to readjust." He cautions against the reckless use of magnets: "Personally, I will err on the side of caution until I am convinced that we know what we are doing."[6] Although Upledger does not cite the abundance of evidence that static magnetic fields are safe, I think that he has a valid point on the issue of the long-term and persistent use of magnets. There has not yet been enough research in this area.

The British National Radiological Protection Board (NRPB) addressed the issue of long-term use when it stated, "There is no direct experimental evidence of any acute, adverse effect on human health due to short-term exposure to static magnetic fields up to about 2T [20,000 gauss]."[7] The emphasis here is on the words "acute" and "short-term."

We simply don't yet know what the long-term effects on the human body are. According to the NRPB, "There is little experimental information on the effects of chronic exposure. So far, no long-term effects have become apparent."[8] In the absence of biological data, the argument at this point comes down to theory. Moulder said, "There is very little theoretical reason to suspect that static fields might cause or contribute to cancer or any other human health problems."[9]

To summarize, the vast majority of scientists see no cause for concern whatsoever regarding side effects and safety issues in magnet therapy. A few practitioners suggest exercising caution, especially with the long-term use of strong magnetic fields. Many practitioners of various forms of medicine are seeing good results with no side effects over time. In countries where magnet therapy has been used for decades, such as Russia and Japan, there is no anecdotal or clinical evidence indicating that magnets are dangerous to health.

As with any form of medicine, you must follow your own instincts and experience. If wearing magnets helps with your pain, the odds are very high that using magnets over time is much less harmful than using anti-inflammatory medication and most probably is not harmful at all. If sleeping on a magnetic mattress pad helps you sleep, then it is probably much better than taking sleeping pills or tossing and turning all night. A few people do exhibit sensitivity to magnets. If you find yourself sensitive to them, but you still want to try magnets, use them for very short periods and remove them as soon as they begin to irritate. The vast majority of people find wearing magnets to be a comfortable experience with beneficial effects.

11

How to Use Magnets

This chapter looks at how to choose, buy, and use magnets. First of all, how do you buy magnets? Is it best to buy them from high street stores, over the Internet, or from multilevel marketing companies? In this chapter, I describe some of the most popular magnetic products currently on the market and how to choose the appropriate types of magnets for different conditions. I then describe how to use these products—where on the body to put them, how long to leave them on, and other relevant concerns. The last part of the chapter examines the confusing and controversial issue of polarities—whether it is best to use north pole, south pole, or bipolar magnets.

BUYING MAGNETS

Let's assume the evidence suggests that magnets may be helpful for your condition and you've decided to give them a try. How do you get hold of them? Which ones are the best? People don't have to have a medical qualification in order to sell magnets, so there is no guarantee that you will be given reliable advice. Although some sellers of magnets are educated about magnet therapy and diligent in their search for useful healing methods, others may be less dependable.

Many of the magnets and magnetic devices on the market today are sold through multilevel marketing companies. This is a mixed blessing. Many salespeople in these companies get involved in selling magnets because they initially had a good personal experience using magnets. This experience makes them enthusiastic, and they can impart all the good news about magnets to you with a certain excitement. They often have a genuine desire to make magnets available to people and to spread the word about this method of therapy. On the downside, these salespeople may not be able to give you the best advice about your particular condition, and they may even tell you things about magnets that are untrue. They don't necessarily do this knowingly; it's more likely that they are either overenthusiastic or misguided in their understanding of what magnets can do. They may have been given incomplete information by their parent company, or they have simply allowed their own zeal to overwhelm their common sense. I have attended large meetings of multilevel marketing companies in which the claims made for magnets were exaggerated and in which the science used to back up these claims was simplistic and often misleading.

The company representatives also have a vested interest in selling you the product, and sometimes this interest can impair their judgment about whether magnets can really be helpful. This said, they probably know much more than the salesperson in your local drug store or retail chain that sells magnetic foot insoles and bargain packs of miscellaneous magnets of different sizes. Also, the magnetic devices sold by the best of the multilevel companies are often superior in quality and design to those sold in chain stores.

I recommend that you look at several types of magnetic devices to get an idea of the quality that is available. However, I do not recommend buying magnets from Web sites without first being able to examine the quality of the products. I know of two Web sites that look okay but that sell magnets of poor quality. Another tip is to look in the clinical studies on magnets for brand names. If doctors have accepted these magnets for their trials, the devices are probably of reliable quality. However, this is not in itself a guarantee, and I would still suggest examining the magnets first, especially if you are buying an expensive product like a mattress pad.

One clear advantage that the multilevel marketing companies offer over catalogs and Web sites is that you have the chance to look over the product before making a purchase, often in the comfort of your own home. On the other hand, all the reputable mail-order companies will give you a refund if their product does not work for you.

The following discussion describes some of the most commonly used products to give you an idea of what type of device might best suit your needs.

MAGNETIC PRODUCTS

All kinds of magnetic products are manufactured these days, ranging from single magnets that you tape to the body to mattress pads filled with magnets to special devices that magnetize water. The most useful and widely used products are described below. The following is not an exhaustive account, so if you don't see the product you need, don't assume that it doesn't exist. The market for magnets is growing every day, and the companies that sell them are constantly inventing and designing new products.

Single Magnets

Commercially available magnets vary in strength from 50 to 10,000 gauss. They come in various sizes, shapes, and configurations to suit different conditions and different parts of the body.

Small, round magnets can be taped securely to acupuncture points or pain trigger points. The best tape to use is the standard adhesive variety designed for the body and available from pharmacy first aid sections. *OMS®* *(Oriental Medical Supply),* the catalog that most professional acupuncturists use, sells tiny magnets—called acu-magnets—that are encased in neat, little circular Band-Aid® adhesive strips, ready to apply to the acupuncture points. These magnets are made from rare earth (a combination of boron, cobalt, and neodymium), a substance that can pick up a great deal of magnetic strength per area in the manufacturing process. This means that although the magnets are tiny, they carry a high gauss rating.[1]

Larger magnets that are not prefitted into a strap or band can also be kept in place with adhesive tape. But unless the magnet is very small, like the ones placed on acupuncture points, keeping it taped in place as you go about your daily life can be frustrating and annoying. This is why wraps and belts with built-in magnets were created—they are so much easier to use. If you do tape a large magnet to your body, and this may be necessary if you have a pain or injury in a place that won't work with any of the wraps, use a wide-band, self-adherent fabric tape, such as the Coban™ brand made by 3M.

Some shapes of magnets can be used without tape. The flat, oblong, credit-card–shaped magnets are convenient for slipping inside a knee or arm bandage. For lower back pain, Nikken makes a back-flex magnet that will stay in place when tucked into the waistband of a pair of pants or a skirt. The back-flex magnet is a large, firm but flexible magnet, about 7 inches long and 5 1/2 inches wide, with two strips of Velcro™ closure material placed lengthwise on the side of the magnet facing away from the skin. The Velcro attaches to the waistband of your underwear or clothing. Users say the back-flex magnet is unobtrusive and comfortable.[2]

Magnetic Wraps

Wraps are available from several companies and come in two main types: those with all the magnets placed in the wrap so that the north pole is on the skin side, and those with alternating north and south poles. Some alternating-pole magnetic devices (such as those manu-factured by Nikken) are arranged in a triangular grid pattern that supposedly enhances the magnetic effect. This type of device does not penetrate the tissue as deeply as a unipolar magnet and, for this reason, is probably best suited to superficial injuries. For injuries that are deeper in the body, such as bone problems or lower-back pain, research is beginning to show that unipolar magnets usually work best. Later in this chap-ter is a discussion that provides more detail about the whole issue of polarities.

As with all other magnetic products, wraps tend to vary in quality. If you are going to wear a wrap often, and if it has a Velcro closure, make sure you get one that is well-made, otherwise it won't last. The only way to damage the magnets themselves is by hitting or drop-ping them, which can disturb the arrangement of the molecules and weaken the magnetic field. So, as long as you treat magnets carefully, they will potentially last forever. However, in a wrap, pad, or similar device, the product will only last as long as the fabric holds up, which is why it is worth buying a well-constructed device made from sturdy materials.

For swollen or injured wrists, a wrist wrap is a use-ful product to invest in. A friend of mine, Sally, is a beautician. She had had swollen painful wrists with seriously inflamed tendons for five years and had tried all kinds of remedies before using a good-quality magnetic wrist wrap. Within the first two days, both wrists were much less sore, and within two weeks, the swelling had gone down so that she was able to see her wrist bones again. There are also similar products specially designed for use on the elbows, hands, knees, thighs, and ankles.

Another friend, Colin, tried a product marketed as a neck wrap. His experience was less successful than Sally's. He has had neck pains for ten years. Although he doesn't appear to have any degeneration of the bone in that area, he suffers periodically from an arthritis-like condition of the cervical vertebrae. He found the wrap rather heavy for his neck and thought that it didn't extend far enough up the neck to be useful. He felt it worked better as a shoulder wrap, as it more fully covered the area. This wrap was an alternating-pole product, with both north and south pole magnets arranged in a triangular grid pattern. With this style of device, the penetration of the magnetism is shallower; therefore, its effectiveness is really limited to the region immediately under the wrap. Obviously, it's important to buy the product that properly covers the area of concern. Colin might have been better off with a unipolar type of magnet, as the magnetic field would have penetrated further into the tissue.

There are also back belts. Here again, find a brand that is well-made and that fits your waist comfortably. If you have to order from a catalog or over the Internet, make sure the company has a return policy if you are not satisfied. A back belt can cost as much as $150, so be sure that you like the feel of it and that it fits correctly. *OMS,* a reliable professional catalog for acupuncturists, chiropractors, medical doctors, and physiotherapists, offers a wide range of back belts and other kinds of wraps.

In most wraps, the magnets are encased in an elastic material that also acts as a supportive bandage for the body part in question. The wrap also keeps that part of the body warm, especially if thermal materials are included in the design. This adds to the therapeutic value of the whole device.

Magnetic Foot Insoles

Magnetic foot insoles are now widely available. I saw some recently in my local drug store, right next to Dr. Scholl's® odor-eaters. Once again, choose your brand with some care. I have not done any consumer testing on these devices, but I imagine that, to some extent, you get what you pay for. People who stand all day at work often find magnetic foot insoles useful and say they have less foot pain during the day.

Magnetic foot insoles also appear to have a particular usefulness for people with diabetes. Dr. Michael Weintraub's study on diabetic peripheral neuropathy (see chapter 8) showed that wearing the insoles was helpful for the pain and tingling of the feet that diabetics sometimes experience.

Many people claim that wearing the insoles makes them feel more energetic. How could this be? From Chinese medicine, we know that there are many acupuncture points in the feet. Foot reflexologists claim that you can treat the whole body by applying pressure to specific parts of the feet that relate to different organs and physiological systems in the body. So it may be that wearing magnetic insoles has some effect on the whole organism.

One friend of mine finds that the insoles help her feel clear and energetic after a day sitting in front of computer equipment. Most creatively, another friend used an insole taped to her thigh to get rid of cellulite. (There's more on these two tales in later chapters.)

There are several different types of insoles. Some are thick and only work in sport-type shoes, others are thinner and suitable for dress shoes, and some have nobbles on the surface that stimulate reflexology points on the sole of the foot.

Magnetic Mattress Pads

Mattresses and mattress pads containing magnets have been popular in Japan for many years and are becoming increasingly popular in the United States. They vary widely in price. For example, *OMS* offers a queen-size, north-pole mattress pad, 75 cm thick, that contains three hundred twenty-four 800-gauss magnets. The pad costs $240 wholesale from the catalog, with a recommended retail value of $325. A fairly basic queen-size pad from MagnaPak costs $490 and contains 366 domino magnets in a $2^{1}/_{2}$ inch foam pad with the north pole uppermost. The deluxe, alternating-pole, Intelli-Rest KenkoPad® by Nikken, made from "memory foam" and covered in high-quality fabric, features "special patented Rubberthane™ nodules for a gentle massaging effect" and retails for $1,500. At the very top end of the market, Nikken sells an actual mattress—not just a pad—complete with the aforementioned Rubberthane nodules, plus "state-of-the-art promo pads [Nikken code for magnets] strategically arranged in the Central Support Zone," all for the princely sum of $1,872 for the queen-size and $2,233 for the king-size, recommended retail price.

When I first started doing research for this book, someone offered to lend me a good-quality mattress pad for a week. In the spirit of research, I thought I should give it a try. The first night I felt overstimulated, and I had a hard time getting to sleep. I woke up at 3:00 A.M. full of energy, but I didn't like the feeling, so I took the pad off the bed. The next night I gave it another try, and this time I put it under my cotton-quilted mattress cover. In retrospect, given what I now know about the penetration of the magnetism from these devices, I wonder if I was getting very much magnetism from the pad at all. Anyway, I found that I then slept very well, and I must say that by the end of the week, I felt I needed less sleep at night—one of the beneficial side effects reported by many mattress pad users.

Since then I have heard numerous stories about the glories of mattress pads. In the summer of 1999, the young tennis player Alexandra Stevenson caused a sensation by getting to the semifinals at Wimbledon. In an interview on NBC, she said that sleeping on a Nikken mattress was a big factor in how well she was playing. Many golfers swear by their magnetic mattress pads and take them on tour.

Hearing all these stories, you can start to get a little blasé. It all begins to merge into one big story. But then you hear something that makes it all come right home. Recently, a friend told me that her aging and much-beloved mother, who has had arthritis for many years, has been sleeping on a magnetic mattress pad for the past couple months. My friend says she can see the bones in her mother's hands for the first time since she can remember.

Magnetic Bracelets and Necklaces

Like mattress pads, magnetic bracelets and necklaces have been popular in Japan for many years and are beginning to be sold in the United States. They are a decorative way of wearing magnets, and most of the magnet distributors feature several magnetic jewelry designs in their catalogs and on their Web sites.

Studies on these products show contradictory results. A study by Dr. Nakagawa, a famous proponent of magnet therapy, reported a decrease of neck and shoulder pain after use of a loose-fitting, magnetically active necklace. But a double-blind study by Hong and associates on the long-term effect of a similar necklace did not find that the necklace generated any significant pain relief.[3] This may be because the intensity of the magnetic fields was rather low in relation to that applied in other studies. In addition, a loose-fitting necklace will not deliver the same focused magnetic energy as will a device that sits directly on either the pain site or an acupuncture point. But some people swear by magnetic jewelry, and there are many anecdotal reports that it can be helpful for people suffering from pain, especially from arthritis.

Products for Magnetizing Water

Reports suggest that magnets can be used to improve the quality of water. When water passes through a magnetic field, the hydrogen ions and dissolved minerals become charged in such a way that the water is softened. There are many anecdotal reports of people who experience healing effects from drinking magnetized water or from using it to wash affected parts of the body. In addition, the softened magnetized water generates less mineralization in water pipes.

There are several products available that are specially designed to attach to water pipes. Or you can simply tape a magnet to the pipes or place a jug of water over a magnet. Opinions vary as to whether the magnet should be south- or north-facing. Apparently plants grow faster when treated with south-magnetized water. If you have a good sense of taste, you can experiment by placing two glasses of water over a magnet of each polarity for fifteen minutes. Then taste the water to determine which you like best. Overall, bipolar treatment appears to be the most widely used. The multisoft water magnets sold by *OMS* are bipolar.

Is there any scientific basis for using magnetized water? You would think that this simple technique would have been studied and that we would have some concrete information by now. Unfortunately, this is not the case, and the lack of decent research makes one suspect that magnetizing water may have limited benefits. A search on the Internet for "magnetized water" brought up 137 results, and 136 of these were references to commercial sites making strong (and often hard-to-believe) claims for the benefits of magnetized water. Only one site mentioned a peer-reviewed, double-blind, placebo-controlled, crossover study. This study was conducted in 1998 at the Medical University of South Carolina's periodontics division and involved 29 subjects. It examined the efficacy of an oral irrigator using magnetized water. The researchers wanted to find out if using the magnetized water in the irrigator had any effect on three parameters: plaque buildup, calculus deposits, and gingival health.

I spoke with Jack Sanders, one of the investigators, who told me that the study was suggested and funded by HydroFloss, a company interested in marketing the irrigation device. The company was inspired to test magnetized water after reading about Russian industrial use of magnetized water. Sanders and his colleagues were extremely skeptical at first and were most surprised by the results of the study. Their results showed that the subjects receiving the magnetized water developed significantly less calculus on their teeth. "Irrigation with magnetized water resulted in 64 percent less calculus compared to the control group."[4] Sanders told me, "We presume this effect occurred because the magnetization changed the ionization of the water."

However, although there was a clinical reduction in gingival inflammation (27 percent lower compared with the control group), this finding was not statistically significant. In addition, there was such minimal effect on the level of bacterial plaque on the teeth that it was not even clinically relevant. Sanders commented,

"The device might be helpful for people who get heavy calculus deposits on their teeth."

To find out more about magnetic technology, I recommend The Cutting Edge Catalog™, which offers a wide range of magnetic technology products.[5]

Wacky Products

At the wacky end of the magnet business, we find companies advertising magnets as the cure for sexual difficulties. One company sells magnets as "Our 'Move Over Viagra' Solution". Their Web site states that magnets "generate heat" (of the thermal variety), one of the ingredients, we are told, of a passionate and romantic evening. (If there's one thing we know about magnets, it's that they don't generate heat.) The Web page goes on to caution the user of this "SuperMagnum" product: "These are very powerful magnets. Until you can gauge your response level and the overall effect they have on you, I recommend that you only wear them for two or three hours at a time, and preferably not in public, lest you find yourself in an embarrassing situation." Such wishful thinking!

Another company markets "sex magnets", called "Vigor Energizing Chips". Again we find more erroneous pseudoscience, including the claim that wearing these magnets will enhance sexual performance and the promise that the product is "lightweight, descreet [sic], optically neutral [!], and washable [thank goodness]".

To be serious for a moment: of course, if magnets could help sexual function, they would be an excellent alternative to medication. Unfortunately, it's quite unlikely that magnets would enhance sexual performance or desire. Magnets do appear to increase blood circulation in certain cases, but this has only been shown when there is some injury to the tissue. Impotence and frigidity are usually caused by deeper systemic problems or by psychological or emotional issues that are not amenable to the wonders of magnetism. A drug like Viagra® can induce blood circulation to the genitals in a powerful way that the humble magnet is unlikely to be able to replicate.

HOW TO USE MAGNETS

Using magnets is really quite simple. To treat painful conditions with magnets, you place the magnet as close as possible to the area that hurts. In addition, you can use trigger points and/or acupuncture points. Trigger points are areas that are very sore. They may be situated on the pain site itself, or they can be in a different part of the body but connected by nerves to the area that hurts. Seventy percent of trigger points coincide with acupuncture points. You can often find trigger points by palpating to determine the most painful spot. If you can't find your pain trigger points by feel alone, there is an atlas of trigger points, written by Travell and Simons (1983). The atlas can help you find which trigger points relate to the site of your pain.

When you place magnets on acupuncture points, you don't need very big magnets and you don't need a lot of depth of magnetic-field penetration. The smallness of the magnets is very convenient. Magnets on acupuncture points can easily be kept on for a period of time. It's best to get a diagnosis from an acupuncturist before putting magnets on points yourself. Find out which acupuncture points are good for you and for your condition and work with those points as instructed. Magnets on acupuncture points have a wider benefit than simply dealing with pain, as they often have a systemic effect as well as a local one. (See chapter 12 for more information on magnets and acupuncture.)

For problems involving large areas of the body, such as lower-back pain, it is probably best to use a wrap device designed to treat a large area while being comfortable to wear. Wearing a large magnet taped to your back all day will probably be an annoyance because it will undoubtedly become untaped and move around beneath your clothing.

When you want to treat the whole body, say in the case of arthritis affecting many joints or fibromyalgia, a magnetic mattress pad may be a good option.

A basic rule of thumb with magnets is the following: magnets either work or they don't. If you don't experience some relief from pain within 15 to 30 minutes, then you probably won't ever experience it with that particular type of magnet on that particular part of the body. When the magnet does work, the effect shows fairly immediately. If you don't get pain relief within 30 minutes, then you probably have the wrong type of magnet or have it on the wrong place on the body, or your condition is simply not amenable to magnet therapy. It doesn't always work. This said, sometimes pain relief will be minimal initially, and over time will become more pronounced. So even a slight reduction in pain is sufficient reason to persist in using the magnet.

The section on polarities further along in this chapter gives more information on how the polarity of the magnet may affect whether it has a therapeutic effect. If you use one type of magnet to no effect, try a different one before you give up on magnets altogether.

How Long Should Magnets Stay On?

If you tape the magnets to your body, you need to take them off periodically for two reasons: first, to keep the tape from irritating the skin, and second, to keep your body from adapting to the magnetic field to the point that the field becomes an ineffective stimulus.

Practitioners vary as to how often they think you should remove the magnets. The acupuncturist Michael Waterhouse (see chapter 12) recommends keeping the magnets on for five days and then leaving them off for two. Other practitioners leave magnets on for longer, although new research suggests that intermittent use is better than continual use. With intermittent use, the body doesn't adapt to the stimulus, which calls into question the value of mattress pads or, at any rate, of sleeping on one every night.

In my interview with Arthur Pilla, he said, "Leaving magnets on all the time is a big mistake. The body starts accommodating to the field and so the magnets start losing effect. It is much better to have intermittent exposure. One hour at a time, repeated two or three times a day, is much better than all the time." Other practitioners have found that you can leave magnets on for longer than Pilla's recommendation, but most agree that periodic removal gives the best results.

When Sally, my beautician friend with the wrist problem, started wearing the wrist wrap, she followed the advice about intermittent use. She slept at night with the wrist wrap on her right wrist, the one that she uses most. During the day, she wore the wrap on her left wrist. This way, she only had to buy one wrap, and the intermittent use on each wrist was better anyway.

POLARITIES

And now, the thorny issue of polarities. The question is: Does it make any difference therapeutically if the north or the south pole of the magnet faces the body? Or should you use a magnetic device that contains magnets in an alternating-polar arrangement, that is, both poles face the body?

Opinions are quite astonishingly heated on this topic. The main debate exists between the scientists and the practitioners. The biophysicists I spoke with were uniform in their opinion that, to date, there is no evidence that using different polarities in treatment makes any difference. Their main interest lies in determining in what ways the magnetic field changes depending on whether alternating poles or single poles are used.

The practitioners, depending on where they trained and who has influenced them, have varying opinions but usually follow the notion that the north pole tends to calm things down, whereas the south pole tends to stimulate. In general, the practitioners agree that there is a difference between the two poles and that it's important to know which pole you are placing next to the body.

Acupuncturists have been influenced by the work of Yushio Manaka, the innovative Japanese acupuncturist who used the following determination of polarity: the north magnetic pole of a magnet is the pole that repels the point of a compass, whereas the south magnetic pole of a magnet is the pole that attracts the point of a compass. This determination is based on the idea that the *geographic* North Pole of the earth is the *geomagnetic* South Pole of the earth. (Dr. Manaka's work is discussed in more detail in chapter 12.)[6] This way of assessing the polarity of magnets has been adopted for general use. It's confusing, to say the least. It suggests that the north pole of a therapeutic magnet behaves like the south pole of a compass needle; that is, the magnet points away from the earth's North Pole. *OMS* sells devices that can help you determine which pole is which.

Dr. William Philpott, following the work of Dr. Roy Davies, has been an influential figure in the development of magnet therapy in the United States. He recommends using only the north pole and thinks that the south pole can be dangerous. Philpott is not in favor with the biophysicists and has never had his research into the biological effects of magnetism published in a peer-reviewed journal. He self-publishes a journal called the *Magnetic Health Quarterly*. (I ordered three issues from American Magnetics and received grainy photocopies of a short and confusing publication at the cost of $30, plus $5 shipping. When the price was quoted to me over the phone, I expected something glossy and full of information. Imagine my surprise when these grim documents of office-copy quality showed up. I'm not sure who is to blame for this blatant rip-off, but it did not endear Dr. Philpott to me. I was left with the impression that his work is as shamefully unprofessional as these poor photocopies masquerading as a reputable journal would suggest.)

Unlike the practitioners, the scientists come to their opinion from their understanding of the way magnets act on tissue and cultures in the lab, as well as from research on animals and humans. Arthur Pilla said, "The idea that one pole is better than another pole is an open question. As a scientist, I have to say that there's no reason to expect that one pole would have a different effect than the other. No one has conclusively shown this. At the laboratory level in lab dishes, there's no difference."

Dr. Marko Markov, the Bulgarian biophysicist who has been researching magnets for thirty years, said:

> Polarity theories such as Philpott's are nonsense. It doesn't make a serious difference which polarity faces the body. This is a different issue than when you have both poles at once on the same side. With bipolar magnets, you have + and − on the same surface. The system has to be very carefully magnetized. Are they effective? They don't penetrate as deeply. They are very convenient for use, but it's possible that they only work for the treatment of superficial problems. The magnetic field in these

devices doesn't penetrate very far, but deep enough
to reach C fibers, which are responsible for the beneficial effects that Dr. Weintraub found in his study.

(For more on Dr. Michael Weintraub's study on diabetic
peripheral neuropathy, see chapter 8.)

Dr. Pilla is currently pursuing research into the
polarity question.

> When you place a magnet on the skin, should you
> have a single pole facing the skin or both poles in a
> geometric pattern? That's not clear at the moment.
> What is clear is that if you have both poles contact-
> ing the skin, you don't get much depth of penetra-
> tion, but you get lots of field gradients right on the
> surface. This may or may not be important; nobody
> knows that yet. When you place a single pole fac-
> ing the skin, you get greater depth of penetration;
> you still get a gradient set up, but it's not as intense
> at the surface.
>
> What is not understood yet is the relationship of
> the geometry of the [magnetic] field to the biologi-
> cal effect. We just don't know that yet. If we took
> the lead from pulsing fields, we would say that it
> probably doesn't matter what the geometry looks
> like as long as the field gets there.

Among practitioners using magnets there is confusion about how to use the two poles. Some say, use the
north pole only; others say, use the north pole to sedate
and calm and the south to excite and stimulate.

There is a developing consensus that using alternating magnets, in which both poles are equally present, works best. Nikken claims to have done extensive
research that supports the use of alternating poles, and
now all their magnetic devices contain magnets of alternating poles. But Nikken refuses to make its research
public, so we can't take this as being reliable advice one
way or the other. The truth is, no one really knows. All

we have to go on is clinical evidence, and there's as much of that to support one argument as another.

Curiously, a similar controversy exists among acupuncturists regarding needle technique. Some schools say that you can tonify (stimulate energy) or sedate (calm and disperse energy) an acupuncture point depending on what is done with the needle. Others say that this is a fallacy and that the body will simply do what it wants once the stimulus of the needle is applied. The tonify/sedate school teaches that if you twirl the needle clockwise, the energy is tonified; if you twirl it counterclockwise, the energy is sedated. This concept sounds very similar to ideas about north and south poles of magnets.

The controversy gets more complicated, just as it does with magnets. Do you leave the needle in, or do you take it out? J. R. Worsley teaches that tonification consists of turning the needle one full circle clockwise, followed by immediate removal of the needle. In his method, sedation is performed by turning the needle one turn counterclockwise and then leaving the needle in place for 30 to 40 minutes. Many other practitioners turn the needle to tonify or sedate and then leave it in, whether or not they are tonifying or sedating. Similarly, there are different ideas about the length of time that magnets should be applied.

In traditional Chinese medicine (TCM, which means acupuncture as it is taught in China today), "even" treatment is recommended, which is neither tonification nor sedation but in between. Even treatment is done by inserting the needle, rotating it back and forth in any direction to find the *chi,* and then leaving the needle in for 30 to 40 minutes or until sufficient change has been noted in the pulses at the wrist. The theory here is that the body will use the influence of the needle in whatever way it needs. Most conditions are a mixture of deficiency and excess, so by this method you avoid the possibility of giving a treatment that is either too stimulating or too sedating. This approach sounds like that of the proponents of bipolar magnets, who say it's the safest method.

Still others say that it is impossible to overtonify or oversedate because the nature of acupuncture is to return the body to homeostasis (normalcy). Similarly, you hear people in the magnet world say that it's impossible to have a bad reaction to magnets because the body will simply no longer accept the stimulus if it's not necessary. This is a very convenient idea and, to my mind, not very believable. In my experience, both acupuncture and magnets can temporarily disturb body energy and, therefore, body health if used in excess and unwisely. Using many very strong magnets for a long time is probably not a good idea, although we really don't know what the outcome might be.

Of course, this disturbance of energy is a relative matter, and possible harm from magnets or acupuncture would not rate along with the side effects or downright poisonous effects of taking the wrong pharmaceutical drug or having unnecessary surgery. I doubt that anyone has actually died as the result of a bad acupuncture treatment or too many magnets. But I do feel that we should take the power of such treatments as acupuncture and magnets seriously. It's too easy to have it both ways—to say that alternative medicine is an effective treatment while at the same time saying it can do no harm. The most logical way of looking at the issue of magnet therapy is to say that any system of treatment that is potent, or that has the power to heal, probably also has the power to damage if used wrongly. At the same time, scary stories about the dangers of using the south pole seem to have little foundation in fact. Magnets, like acupuncture, are a relatively benign healing tool and can be used with confidence.

For the time being, the polarity issue remains unanswered. There is a wealth of clinical evidence from practitioners, mostly acupuncturists, that polarity makes a difference. There is also a good deal of anecdotal evidence from people using alternating magnetic pole products (such as those manufactured by Nikken) with great success.

If you are using an alternating-pole product and feel no effect, you would be well-advised to try a unipolar magnet instead. As already discussed, the alternating-pole, or bipolar, magnets don't seem to penetrate as deeply into the tissue, so they are often less effective than single-pole magnets for certain conditions, particularly deep-seated pain in the hips and lower back.

A study published in the *Journal of the American Medical Association* in March 2000 found no evidence of therapeutic effect on chronic lower back pain. The study used alternating-pole magnets, which are not always the device of choice for this condition.

With the type of magnet employed by the study, the depth of penetration is not sufficient to get an adequate dose of magnetic field at the target tissue. To achieve an adequate dose in the lumbar area, the magnetic field would need to penetrate at least 1 inch (25 mm) below the skin. The researchers misleadingly list the magnetic field at 300 gauss, but this measurement refers to a particular point on the surface of the magnet. The magnetic field from bipolar magnets falls to negligible levels at about 5 mm from the magnet surface, so the researchers' observation of no effect is not surprising. If, in addition to the sham control group, the researchers had included a third control group using a unipolar magnet with the north pole facing the skin and a fourth control group using the south pole facing the skin, different and more meaningful results might have been achieved.[7]

There were several other aspects of the study design that also rendered it unconvincing in its conclusions. As a result, this study, which appears to nullify the usefulness of magnets for back pain, is essentially flawed.

SUMMARY

In conclusion, for minor conditions such as sprains and soft tissue injuries, you can probably use magnets by yourself, assisted by the advice contained in this chapter. For more complex conditions involving any kind of long-term or serious health issue, it may be wise to seek the advice of a professional experienced with using magnet therapy. Chapters 12 and 13 explain how various practitioners in several disciplines are using magnet therapy at this time.

12

Magnets and Acupuncture

As we saw in chapter 2, there has been a long association between Oriental medicine and the therapeutic use of magnets. Still, today, in the broad field of alternative and complementary medicine, acupuncturists are the most likely to be knowledgeable about magnet therapy. This chapter shows how acupuncture and magnets fit together in both philosophical and practical terms.

For at least two thousand years, acupuncture has been recognized as a highly effective system of medicine in China and elsewhere in the East. During the past two decades, it has become increasingly accepted in the West. Official organizations, such as the National Institutes of Health (NIH) and the World Health Organization (WHO), recognize acupuncture as a useful therapeutic system. The NIH Web page refers to acupuncture as "one of the oldest, most commonly used medical procedures in the world. Research shows that acupuncture is beneficial in treating a variety of health conditions."

As early as 1979, the World Health Organization, the health branch of the United Nations, recognized acupuncture as a viable, inexpensive method of health care and recommended that governments put funds into research and into creating acupuncture clinics. The WHO lists more than 40 conditions for which acupuncture may be used.[1] In 1993, the FDA estimated that

Americans made 9 to 12 million visits per year to acupuncture practitioners and spent as much as $500 million on acupuncture treatments.[2] In 1995, an estimated 10,000 nationally certified acupuncturists were practicing in the United States. That number was expected to double by the year 2000. About a third of certified acupuncturists in the United States are also medical doctors.[3]

WHAT ACUPUNCTURE SHOWS US ABOUT MAGNETS

It's worth taking the time to look at both the theoretical basis of acupuncture and the current scientific understanding of how it works. This information may give us some clues about how magnets work. Although conventional science is still scratching its head about how magnets are helping people's pain and inflammation, Chinese medicine offers some hints. Sometimes it helps to look at a phenomenon from a new set of criteria and through the lens of a different paradigm.

Traditional Chinese Acupuncture Theory

Acupuncture is based on the fundamental concept of *chi*. To understand acupuncture, you first have to grasp the idea of chi and, for the moment, accept that it exists. The term "chi" is not directly translatable into English, but broadly speaking, it means energy. (*Energy* itself is a word that has become used increasingly in recent years and for which the definitions are rather foggy.) Chi moves through the body along channels called meridians. It connects the outside of the body with the structural system and the internal organs and is responsible for the health of not only the physical body, but also the mind, emotions, and spirit.

In a state of health, chi streams freely through the meridians, infusing the body with vitality and creating a wholeness of body, mind, and spirit. The body is strong and resistant to disease; the mind is clear and manifests a steady intelligence; emotions flow freely and appropriately; the heart is loving, spontaneous, and joyful; and the spirit is connected to the heavens at all times. In Chinese thinking, human beings are the connectors between earth and heaven. Through careful stewardship of the physical realm, and through paying attention to the word of the heavens, human beings can live in harmony with the rest of life.

Disharmony of body, mind, or spirit can result from an imbalance of various factors. The primary factor is the relative balance of *yin* and *yang,* the two polar, yet complementary, forces that in Chinese thinking represent the essential polarity that generates and expresses life. This polarity manifests in nature as masculine and feminine, light and dark, sun and moon, inside and outside, hot and cold, full and empty. It also manifests as the north pole and the south pole of a magnet. When yin and yang are balanced, chi flows clearly, and the body, mind, and spirit are healthy.

When chi fails to flow correctly, several things can happen. Sometimes poor diet, difficult external physical conditions, emotional neglect, genetic tendencies, or infectious illness result in the supply of chi being diminished. When this happens, there is not enough chi to nourish the whole body, mind, and spirit for overall health to be maintained. Over time, such deficiencies of chi cause generalized problems as the whole system becomes weakened.

In many cases, there is sufficient chi, but it gets stuck and builds up in one part of the body. This stagnation can cause many symptoms such as pain, swelling, and congestion, which in turn can lead to many kinds of diseases. Chi blocks occur because of injury—physical, emotional, or spiritual. In the Chinese system, the body, mind, emotions, and spirit are all interconnected. For example, the brain is connected to the kidneys and is the seat of certain kinds of cognition, the heart is responsible for the sense of joy, and the liver is responsible for the health of the emotions in general. A stagnant liver (all too common these days) results in an inability to express emotions freely and appropriately. Chi blocks can also be caused by emotional repression. In Chinese medicine, cause and effect are more conjoined than they are in Western thought.

How you think about a situation, how you express yourself, and how much you can stay loving in the midst of difficulty are all functions of different organs in the body, which work together and influence each other. In a state of health, all these organs, functions, and meridians work together like the different instruments in an orchestra. They are all essential, and they are all connected. If one part of the body is weakened or the chi becomes congested, it affects other parts in a clearly defined set of relationships that was identified by Chinese doctors at least two thousand years ago.

In Chinese medicine, you can treat a person before he or she actually manifests symptoms and becomes sick. There are diagnostic methods, such as a special way of taking the pulse at the wrist, that function as early warning signs of impending illness. Either as a preventative method or when illness has already manifested, acupuncture is used to balance yin and yang and to unblock the flow of energy. In this way, the health of the body, mind, and spirit is restored. In addition, several other traditional Chinese medicine practices, including tai chi, chi gong, and herbal medicine, can be used to improve the flow of chi.

Scientific Understanding of Acupuncture

Conventional science has yet to identify acupuncture meridians or to measure or "see" chi. Some researchers speculate that meridians are located throughout the body's connective tissue.[4] Others do not believe that chi exists at all.[5] In general, acupuncturists tend not to be troubled by this controversy. For them, the effect is proof enough that meridians and chi exist. Acupuncture has been tried and tested by time, and ultimately, there is no better proof than that. However, the discovery of the mechanism by which acupuncture works will be a breakthrough for science and for medicine in general.

Some aspects of the acupuncture puzzle have already become clear. In the light of our quest to understand magnet therapy, it is interesting to note that much of the study on acupuncture so far has focused on how it alleviates pain. This research has revealed a whole new realm of knowledge about the mechanisms of natural pain relief in the body. It has helped us understand how acupuncture stimulates the body's natural ability to deal with pain and inflammation.

Scientists currently believe that stimulation of acupuncture points causes the central nervous system (the brain and spinal cord) to release chemicals into the muscles, spinal cord, and brain. It is not known exactly how this mechanism operates, although there are several theories (see below). These chemicals—primarily endorphins and enkephalins—have the function of changing the experience of pain. In addition, the release of these hormones causes a chain reaction, provoking the release of other chemicals, such as hormones, that affect the body's self-regulating systems. It is thought that this chain of biochemical changes stimulates the body's natural healing capacity.[6]

How does stimulation of an acupuncture point do this? There are several mechanisms that are currently understood to play a part in this complex dance. Studies show that acupuncture points are conductors of electromagnetic signals. It has been relatively easy to demonstrate that resistance to electrical stimulus is lower at the site of the points than at the surrounding tissue. Electromagnetic signals in the body are currently understood to be minute electrical impulses that transmit information through and between nerve cells. For example, electromagnetic signals convey information about pain and other sensations within the body's nervous system.[7]

Stimulation of acupuncture points causes electromagnetic signals to be relayed at a greater rate than under normal conditions. These signals appear to stimulate the flow of naturally occurring substances in the body that act as painkillers, such as endorphins. The signals also appear to activate immune system cells that are specific for the area in the body that is injured or diseased.[8,9]

The brain secretes natural substances that behave like opiates. These substances, called opioids or endorphins, cause a sense of well-being and diminish pain. Opioids are made by a group of nerve cells in the brain. They relax muscles, dull pain, and reduce cardiovascular workloads. Morphine and other opiate drugs affect these same nerve cells. It has been known for about 20 years that certain experiences stimulate the production of natural opioids. The bodily and emotional satisfaction felt after doing strenuous exercise, having sex, completing an arduous task, even clearing one's desk of extraneous paperwork, is caused by the release of opioids.

During acupuncture treatments, research shows that several types of opioids are released into the central nervous system.[10] This release accounts not only for the reduction in pain experienced by acupuncture patients, but also for the deep sense of peaceful relaxation that so many people feel by the end of a treatment.

The release of endorphins into the bloodstream during an acupuncture treatment has also been shown to reduce blood pressure and to allow the heart to pump less strenuously.[11]

Studies suggest that acupuncture affects brain chemistry in a beneficial way by altering the release of neurotransmitters and neurohormones. In addition, acupuncture has been shown to influence the areas of the central nervous system that govern sensation and involuntary body functions. Such functions include immune responses and the autonomic regulation of blood pressure, blood flow, and body temperature.[12,13]

Pain Relief, Acupuncture, and Magnetic Resonance Imaging

In a curious confluence of science, where magnets, acupuncture, and modern scientific method converge, we now have further proof that the ancient Chinese system of healing works to reduce pain. A new imaging technique developed from MRI technology has helped us to understand how acupuncture works and has confirmed that acupuncture does, indeed, cause measurable changes in the body.

The new technique is called functional magnetic resonance imaging (fMRI) and was used in a study performed on 12 patients during 1999 at the University of Medicine and Dentistry of New Jersey in Newark. The fMRI was used to measure pain activity in the brain. Dr. Huey-Jen Lee, the lead author of the study, explained that areas of the brain light up during fMRI, measuring increased blood flow in the part of the brain being stimulated.

When you are in pain, your brain activity increases. Conversely, a pain-relieving therapy results in decreased brain activity. Dr. Lee wanted to see if applying acupuncture would result in lowered brain activity, and he used the fMRI to measure this. First, all 12 subjects were tested for their brain response to pain. A thin electrical metal rod was placed on the inside and outside of the subjects' upper lips. All the subjects showed marked brain activity in response to the pain produced by the electrical current.

Seven subjects were then given acupuncture in the Hegu point (Co4), situated in the web between the thumb and forefinger on the back of the hand. This is a major point in Chinese medicine for controlling pain, especially of the head, face, and neck. After 30 minutes of having the needle inserted, the brains of the seven subjects were scanned, and the fMRI showed that four out of the seven had far less brain activity; these four also subjectively reported that they felt much less pain. In the remaining five patients, Lee combined electricity with acupuncture to even greater effectiveness. All five showed decreased brain activity.

In this technique, called electroacupuncture, electrical stimulus is applied to the acupuncture needles. Some practitioners report increased pain-relief capacity from combining electrical stimulus with needling. The study confirmed this clinical experience.[14]

Conditions Treated by Acupuncture

It is now widely accepted that acupuncture is a useful therapy for a wide range of conditions. As mentioned earlier, the WHO has a list of 40 conditions for which acupuncture is recommended. In November 1997, the NIH convened a panel of scientists, researchers, and practitioners to discuss acupuncture. They found that studies supported the use of acupuncture for nausea caused by surgical anesthesia and cancer chemotherapy, for post-surgical dental pain, for stroke rehabilitation, and for treating addiction, headaches, menstrual cramps, tennis elbow, fibromyalgia, myofascial pain, osteoarthritis, lower-back pain, carpal tunnel syndrome, and asthma.[15] You'll notice that many of these conditions are also on the list of conditions for which people are finding magnet therapy helpful. And just as with magnet therapy, Americans seek acupuncture treatment mainly to relieve chronic pain, especially of the lower back or caused by arthritis.[16,17,18]

THE DEVELOPMENT OF MAGNET THERAPY BY ACUPUNCTURISTS

Ancient Chinese doctors understood that magnets had curative properties and used them to heal wounds, relieve pain and arthritis, strengthen the kidneys and bones, and enhance hearing and sight. In Chinese medical thinking, magnets work like acupuncture in that they affect the circulation of chi.

Although the Chinese have used magnets therapeutically for at least two thousand years, they have emphasized the use of needles and herbs more. In Japan, the therapeutic use of magnets has become more sophisticated, largely due to the pioneering work of the remarkable Yushio Manaka, who was one of the great Japanese acupuncturists of the twentieth century. Manaka did a great deal to synthesize modern knowledge of physics with ancient Eastern knowledge of energy.

Manaka adapted Western systems theory and information theory in order to describe and inform the traditional Eastern medical worldview. In his model, chi becomes information and the meridians become information channels; yin-yang and the five elements (another classification of chi) become signals systems with low energy content and high information content. Specific acupuncture points are receptor sites for specific signal inputs.[19]

Manaka developed his theories by doing many experiments. As a physicist as well as a doctor of acupuncture, he was very intrigued by the possibilities of using magnets therapeutically. He was able to show that acupuncture points are susceptible to influence from very subtle stimuli, such as magnets, as well as from the stronger stimuli of needles and moxibustion (a technique in which burning herbs are used to send heat into the acupuncture point).[20]

Manaka developed several tools and gadgets, including ion-pumping cords (sometimes referred to as ion-transfer cords). These cords link a needle in one acupuncture point to another needle in another point. He originated this method in the 1940s as a treatment for burns and found it to be very useful. He theorized that when placed correctly, the cord conducted positive ions away from the burn. Later, he developed specific treatments that use these cords for many conditions with great effectiveness.

The ion-pumping cord device is interesting in the context of magnet therapy because it probably works by conducting magnetic energy from one part of the body to another. In addition, some practitioners use the cords with magnets instead of needles. The cords are made from copper wire or silver chain containing a germanium or silicone diode.

According to Manaka, "The cord can act as an antenna for electromagnetic fields and converts these magnetic fields into a small current that flows in only one direction, according to the orientation of the diode."[21] Manaka found that if the subject was placed in a Faraday cage and shielded from normal background electromagnetism, treatment with the cords did not work. He freely admits that he could not explain all of the results of his experiments, and the exact mechanism by which the ion-pumping cords work has yet to be understood.

Another Japanese scientist, Tada Kono, showed that there are specific abdominal reflex points that worsen or improve the tone of the abdominal muscles when north or south magnets are applied to them.[22] Other Japanese acupuncturists, such as Osamu Ito, have further refined the use of magnets, developing treatment protocols for conditions that are usually difficult to treat.

There has also been considerable interest in electromagnetism and acupuncture in Germany. Most notable is the work of Rheinhold Voll, who developed a method of diagnosis by measuring the electrical charge at certain acupuncture points.

The American Association of Oriental Medicine (AAOM) sponsors lectures for students and features a lecture on magnet therapy. Most of this lecture focuses on which acupuncture points to apply the magnets to, just like a lecture on acupuncture technique using needles, although the combinations of points are sometimes slightly different. The most recent AAOM lecture on magnets included point combinations for menstrual problems, fibroid tumors, and cancer prevention. (In Chinese medicine, cancer is seen as a disease that originates with chi stagnation and that can be treated before a tumor actually develops.)

HOW ACUPUNCTURISTS USE MAGNETS

In chapter 1, we met Sarah, who received magnet therapy at her acupuncturist's office. Her experience was fairly typical, although acupuncturists vary to some extent in the way they use magnets. I spoke with six experienced acupuncturists who described in detail their methodology and clinical experience with magnets. The following descriptions should give you some idea of what to expect if you go to an acupuncturist for magnet therapy.

Michael Waterhouse is a licensed acupuncturist in the state of California and has been a practicing acupuncturist for more than 20 years. He trained in England and China and was dean of the California Acupuncture College for several years. He has a clinic in Beverly Hills and is a clinical instructor at the UCLA School of Medicine. He is the first non-M.D. acupuncturist to have hospital privileges at a major teaching hospital.

> I began using magnets on my patients about three or four years ago. When I first heard about them, I have to say that I was skeptical, but I thought that there was some physiological basis that made sense to me. I was familiar with Becker's work, and I could see how the magnetic force could influence the healing power of the body.

Robert Becker, author of *The Body Electric: Electromagnetism and the Foundation of Life* and *Cross-Currents: The Perils of Electropollution, The Promise of Electromedicine,* was one of the first scientists to discover the tiny electrical currents generated by bone when it is healing. This discovery led him to develop the use of electromagnetism in healing nonunion fractures and to become a pioneer in the field of bioelectromagnetics. His theories and understanding of the subtle levels at which electromagnetism can both heal and harm have been very influential on medical practitioners working with magnetic energy.

In the early 1970s, intrigued by the reports of acupuncture-induced anesthesia brought back by members of President Nixon's trip to China, Becker measured the electrical characteristics of the meridians and the acupuncture points. The places where resistance was lower showed up at the same places on all the people tested. These places corresponded exactly to the acupuncture points. According to Becker, "Our readings also indicated that the meridians were conducting current, and . . . showed a flow into the central nervous system."[23]

Becker's work was important for acupuncturists. As Michael Waterhouse commented,

> Becker's work showed that there was a scientific basis to acupuncture, that it works by exerting a weak bioelectrical force that normalizes the body's own low-amperage current.
>
> When you stimulate an acupuncture point by needles, laser, ultrasound, thumb pressure, or heat, the stimulus has both a systemic and a local effect. If all of these stimuli generate such an effect, why not magnets? Acupuncture essentially works on a homeostatic principle. It encourages normal functioning to return, and I assume that with magnets the same rule applies.
>
> When people came in with little aches and pains, I tried taping a magnet on the area of pain and sending them home with instructions to leave it on all the time for five days. I would put a little round magnet on an aching finger, or stuff magnets inside a wristband for wrist pain. I would do acupuncture as normal, and then put the magnets on the area of pain.
>
> I found that using magnets in this way appeared to speed up the healing process. These days I use 800-gauss, gold-plated magnets from Japan mostly, and occasionally credit-card–size magnets for an area like the knee. In fact, that was one of the first experiences that got me interested in magnets. I had knee surgery myself and thought I might as well try slipping a credit-card–size magnet inside my bandage. I kept it on for two weeks nonstop, and I found that it accelerated the healing process and caused a reduction in pain.
>
> More recently I've started using magnets on acupuncture points. For example, for a patient with heat in the stomach [a classical Chinese diagnosis: symptoms may include gastritis, stomach

pain, ulcers], I'll tape a magnet onto Stomach 41 [a point on the foot classically used to drain heat from the stomach]. It's harder to tell in these cases exactly what effect the magnets are having because I'm also using herbs and acupuncture. I assume that, like acupuncture, the magnet helps to normalize the body's energy.

Phil Caylor is a licensed acupuncturist in the state of California and has a clinic in Santa Cruz. He has been using magnets for more than ten years. He mostly uses magnets with patients who don't like needles. He puts the magnets on the same part of the body where he would put acupuncture needles. He tapes a 9,000-gauss magnet (gold, from *OMS*) over the point for half an hour, always using the north pole of the magnet facing the body. At the end of the 30-minute session, he exchanges the powerful magnet for a 600-gauss magnet, which stays on the patient for a week until the next treatment.

Caylor said, "If the patient keeps the 9,000-gauss magnet for too long, it can cause a too-rapid detoxification, which can give rise to severe headaches." Caylor told me that he has used magnets with great success on migraine headaches, premenstrual syndrome, digestive problems, colds, and flu, as well as for speeding the healing of injuries. Unlike some other practitioners of acupuncture and otherwise, Caylor hasn't found a limit to the conditions that magnets can help:

> If the person responds to magnets, then they work well on pretty much anything the person may have. Overall, I think that needles are probably more effective because they go straight to the point, but I find that magnets work really well. They stimulate the points just like a needle or heat would. And on some people, magnets even work better.

We met **Agatha Colbert** in chapter 6. She is the author of the study published in February 2000 that shows that sleeping on magnetic mattress pads can help people with fibromyalgia. Dr. Colbert, an M.D. who mainly practices acupuncture, said:

> My practice is now about 95 percent acupuncture. It's very satisfying work. One reason I use magnets on acupuncture points is that I see a lot of children in my practice, and they tend to dislike needles. When I found that acu-magnets were as effective in children as needle acupuncture, I began to use magnets as an alternative to needles in adults and found that the treatments were very successful.
>
> Depending on the patient's condition and preference, I use either magnets or needles. If the patient is afraid of needles, I'll use magnets during the first treatment. After getting a sense of how the patient responds, I might then add needles or continue to use magnets alone. For some individuals, needles are more effective. If a person feels strongly that magnets are not enough, I am more inclined to use needles. Some patients are very responsive to magnetic energy. There are people who do not need needles, and others that do. It is nice to have options.
>
> I also use larger body magnets for pain conditions. This is a good self-help technique. I do a combination of teaching people how to use magnets themselves and of using them in the actual treatment.
>
> We don't know enough about magnet strength yet. There's presumably a window of magnetic-field polarity, strength, frequency, and duration of use that will enhance healing better than another, but clinical research is insufficient at this stage to give us an answer to this question. Dr. Marko Markov's work [a Bulgarian biophysicist working in the United States] shows that between 200 and

600 gauss delivered to the target tissue has the most effect.

I often send the patient home with magnets on the point that was needled during the treatment. I tape a little tiny circular low-gauss magnet and tell the patient to leave it on for the week.

Colbert studied magnet therapy with Kiiko Matsumoto, an innovative doctor of Oriental medicine whose work is influenced by the legacy of Yushio Manaka. From Dr. Matsumoto, Colbert learned about using the ion-pumping cords invented by Dr. Manaka. Colbert has adapted this method to enable patients to treat themselves at home.

> My background is in rehab medicine. I believe that home therapy is really important. If somebody is interested in doing a home program, I determine which points they need, and if those points are conducive to using ion-pumping cords and magnets, I'll teach them how to do that. They'll do that every day for 20 to 30 minutes at home on their own. That's the piece that I really enjoy because it lets them treat themselves. It saves them a lot of money and time. Acupuncture is so time-consuming and expensive. And in the West, it's usually just not practical for people to have treatments more often than once a week. For many conditions in China, you'd have a treatment every day or every other day.
>
> The goal is to change the electromagnetic field of the body so that the body's built-in healing mechanisms are encouraged to operate. The results of doing a home program with magnets may take a little longer than would occur with daily needling but will eventually have the same beneficial effect. For people with chronic illnesses, and that is generally the population coming for acupuncture, this approach works well. I first tried this method with

an attorney who had diverticulitis. He was a very diligent patient, and so I sent him off with instructions, the magnets, and the ion-pumping cords. He came back two months later having done it every day, and his symptoms had improved significantly.

In the clinic, I also use an electromagnetic machine with 2,000- to 3,000-gauss magnets for a stronger effect, for people who need a more powerful energetic input. I choose to use magnets for several reasons. First, if the patient wants them. Second, if I want to use a pair of points that lend themselves to the ion-pumping cord method. Third, magnets are relatively inexpensive. And fourth, they work.

Colbert uses 10,000-gauss magnets and has people apply those at home for 20 to 30 minutes with the ion-pumping cords once a day. According to Colbert, "I have [patients] come in to see me within a couple of weeks to see how it's going. Some conditions, such as kidney deficiency or blood stagnation, take a long time, say three to four months, before results are seen."

Dr. Colbert is currently designing a study to see how magnets worn in the top of a baseball cap can help with the treatment of depression. This technique is based on a traditional Chinese formula for treating depression, which involves putting several needles in special points *(Sishencong)* on the top of the head.

James Moran is a certified acupuncture physician in the state of Massachusetts and has been working with magnets for the past fifteen years. Like Dr. Colbert, he favors the ion-pumping cords and was trained by Kiiko Matsumoto. Moran, whom we met in chapter 8, was one of the authors of the study on premature babies.

In his practice, Moran works with static magnets alone and also with static magnets and ion-pumping cords. He has used the technique of combining magnets with the ion-pumping cords on many patients with chronic fatigue, as well as on those with chemical sensitivity and candidiasis.

> These people had already had acupuncture, and it seemed that the softer treatment with the magnets and the ion-pumping cords had a better effect. I use Hara diagnosis [a special way of palpating the abdomen] and reflexology to get feedback about the treatment. When treating the deepest layer of energy, which is where you have to get to with these conditions, you see a corresponding reflex level change. I've been evolving this method of treatment using magnets for 15 years.
>
> I use the north-facing pole. I find that this works best. I don't agree with the alternating-field magnets. In line with Philpott's work, I am sure that the body wants a north field. I think that the alternating-polarity magnets give the body a message that it will eventually ignore. It's too confusing for the body.

Holly Guzman is a licensed acupuncturist in the state of California, with a practice in Santa Cruz. She uses magnets widely in her practice. Like James Moran and Agatha Colbert, Guzman also studied with Kiiko Matsumoto, the well-known Japanese acupuncturist who has specialized in the use of magnets for many years. Guzman has also gathered an abundance of notes from classes in China and Japan. Her notes show that there are doctors in those countries who are experimenting extensively with the use of magnets on a wide range of conditions, from digestive disturbances to diabetes to psychological problems.

Guzman finds that magnets are more effective than other therapies for several conditions. She always uses magnets when there is bone pain and arthritic pain from old injuries, for accelerating the healing of fractures to cracked ribs, and for healing scar tissue. Guzman told me, "Magnets are very effective for helping the healing of scar tissue, even old scarring." She uses magnets in combination with specific acupuncture points for conditions involving structural imbalance, such as scoliosis, and certain groups of symptoms, such as inner knee pain and stomach problems.

Diane Black is a licensed acupuncturist in the state of California with a practice in Santa Monica.

> I was introduced to the concept of magnets about 10 years ago. I treat a lot of children and young people in my practice, and many of them are needle-phobic, [as are] a few adults. I started experimenting with using magnets instead of needles. I could tell it was working by using the feedback from the patients who would say, "Oh, I really feel the energy moving." Of course, that's not an objective measurement, but I have other methods to gauge the success of the treatment. I take note of the changes in the pulse, and I also practice a system called manual thermal diagnosis. With this technique, you scan the thermal field, and you can check for how well the treatment is going. For example, say there was heat in the liver before, and now, after the treatment, the heat has dissipated.
>
> I don't like the ion-pumping cords, because generally my approach is to activate the body's own capacity to heal itself, and the ion pump is more directive than that. It says the body must use the energy this way.
>
> I use the magnets on the points just as if [I were doing] a needle treatment. I use the north pole toward the body. I studied with Michael Tierra a year ago, and since then I've been using the 9,000-gauss gold magnets, and I've found them to be incredibly effective for acute back pain and acute knee pain.

I also do auricular therapy [ear points], using the little magrain magnets, the size of a dot, specially designed for use in the ear. I use them for stop-smoking treatment on the lung point, *shen men,* and sympathetic nervous system, and often adrenal as well.

I know there's a controversy about the polarities, so I tried them out on myself. I had a problem with my knee, and when I put the south pole on, the knee swelled up and felt warmer and more congested. When I put the north pole on, the swelling went down.

I've seen good results from the alternating-field magnetic products, too. I have a patient who had a large keloid scar on her chest, which has almost gone away since sleeping on a magnetic mattress pad. Another patient had sprained her ankle four times in a year. I gave her a magnetic ankle wrap to wear while she was skiing, and she has not sprained her ankle since.

Diane Black also practices a technique called visceral manipulation.

I've found that putting magnets on an area after doing a manipulation seems to extend the life of the treatment. For example, if I tape a magnet to CV14 [a point on the upper abdomen] after I've adjusted a hiatal hernia, the treatment lasts longer.

So yes, in my experience, treatment with magnets can be very effective. It takes longer. A single treatment using magnets takes around 40 minutes, instead of 20 to 30 minutes with a needle. I think this is because it takes longer for the magnet to start attracting the chi. With a needle, you, the acupuncturist, call the chi and then stimulate it. With the magnet, there's a period of time while the magnet is gradually attracting the chi.

SUMMARY

The examples of acupuncturists described in this chapter show that there is a range of ways of working with magnets. As acupuncturists gain experience using magnets, they often become increasingly sophisticated in the way they use them.

Magnets are also being used in conjunction with other forms of therapy. In chapter 13 I describe how various practitioners are finding magnets to be useful adjuncts to their respective types of therapy.

13

Using Magnets
with Other Therapies

Magnet therapy is often most effective when combined with other remedies. In addition, when you choose to have magnet therapy with another method of treatment, you will usually be under the guidance of a medical professional, which, as discussed in chapter 11, has several advantages.

WHY COMBINE MAGNETS
WITH OTHER THERAPIES?

The combination of therapies adds to the efficacy of each. For example, combining magnets with herbal remedies means that a far greater range of conditions can be treated. The organs and internal systems of the body are nourished by the herbs at the same time as the exterior is stimulated by the magnets. In Chinese medicine, serious and long-term conditions are usually treated with a combination of herbs and acupuncture for the same reason.

Magnets can be combined with any therapy, providing the patient does not have a condition that is contraindicated for magnet therapy, such as pregnancy. Chapter 12 examined in detail how acupuncturists work with magnets. This chapter examines some of the other systems of medicine in which magnets or magnetic remedies are becoming popular, including herbalism, homeopathy, body work, dentistry, and conventional medicine.

MAGNETS AND HERBAL MEDICINE

The chief pioneer in the field of magnets and herbal medicine is Michael Tierra, author of *Biomagnetic and Herbal Therapy*. Tierra is a doctor of Chinese medicine, naturopathy, and herbalism. Like many practitioners, both conventional and alternative, Tierra first became intrigued by the therapeutic properties of magnets when he used them on an injury of his own.

> The elbow pain originated from an unknown cause, perhaps an injury or strain. It had persisted for at least two weeks; during that time I tried acupuncture and herbal treatments, which offered only minor temporary relief. As is well known, soft tissue injuries can take some time for repair.
>
> I decided to experiment with magnets to treat the problem. While I had previously heard of magnet therapy, I had no personal experience or further knowledge of its use. When I taped a small 10,000-gauss acuband magnet directly on the skin over the center of the pain in my arm, I was amazed to find that the pain almost entirely disappeared within five minutes.[1]

Tierra went on to do a series of experiments on himself to determine how to use the magnets most effectively. "I discovered that when the south side of the magnet was against the skin, the pain intensified, and by reversing the magnet to north [the pain] was alleviated."[2]

Tierra's long experience with magnets has made him an enthusiastic proponent: "I have found biomagnetic therapy to be approximately 90 percent effective for the relief of pain and conditions caused by inflammation."[3] Conditions that he has treated with success include colitis and other gastrointestinal complaints, arthritis, acute and chronic lower back pain, asthma, upper respiratory allergies, and migraines.

> Now, with the expanded methods of application using magnetized water, magnetized oils, magnetic mattresses, jewelry, and so forth, I am convinced that there is no condition for which biomagnetic therapy would not be at least helpful.[4]

Tierra's book includes treatment protocols for specific conditions combining herbs and magnet therapy. For example, for liver diseases, such as hepatitis and jaundice, he recommends placing a north or bipolar magnet over the right hypochondriac region (just below the lower rib on the right side of the body) and drinking south-magnetized water. In addition, the patient should take a mixture of dandelion root, milk thistle seed, wild yam, barberry root, and fennel seed.[5]

Following is an example of a case in which magnets were used with herbs to great effect. Once again, this story came to me when a colleague called me about an unrelated work issue and we got chatting. When I told her I was writing a book on magnet therapy, she told me about her very successful experience using a combination of magnets and herbs to treat cellulite on her thigh.

Sabrina is a Toronto-based writer and editor. She spends a great deal of time indoors, due to her work, the Canadian climate, and the long winters. When Sabrina was in her mid-thirties, she developed severe cellulite along the outside of one of her thighs. Many women suffer from unsightly cellulite, and it is considered medically untreatable—a common problem that affects women as they age. Men rarely get cellulite, for reasons not yet understood. There are all kinds of expensive treatments offered by cosmetics companies and other outfits, but Sabrina felt they were too expensive and also unlikely to offer any lasting cure. Instead, she cleverly figured out a way to heal her cellulite using a magnetized foot insole.

> I had read a book by Leslie Kenton called *The Cellulite Revolution,* in which she talks about cellulite as a health issue to do with toxicity, not just an aesthetic issue. She says that cellulite is caused by a build up of toxins in lymph and other tissues of the leg.
>
> Then I noticed that along with the cellulite, I was also getting some spider veins in that area of my leg, so I figured it was time to do something about my circulation. I thought, I'm only 37; if my circulation doesn't improve, I'm going to be in trouble, so I'd better see if I can deal with this before it gets any worse.
>
> In addition to looking awful, the cellulite hurt. I had almost constant pain on the outside of my thigh. The cellulite was all along the outside of my left thigh, along the gall bladder meridian [one of the acupuncture channels along which chi is said to flow]. There was one patch that looked like an orange peel and the rest of it looked like marbled paper—big patches with rivulets between them. It was limited in area and painful.
>
> I had had it for a couple of months before I began to try to heal it. I thought of magnets because I had been told that they stimulate circulation. I thought, well, if the circulation is poor in that part of my thigh, perhaps a magnet will help. So at night I would put on a leg warmer and slip a magnetized foot insole into it so that it lay against my thigh, along the area that had the most cellulite.

After the first night, when I woke up, I saw that my thigh had become slightly hot, puffy, and reddish.[6] I knew the magnet was doing something. I continued to use it on a regular basis, and sometimes I would wear it all night and all day. Pretty soon there was no pain in the area, and I noticed that the skin was getting less lumpy.

I had been using the magnet for about two weeks, with noticeable gradual improvement, when I found out that yarrow, the herb, is really good for circulation and helps the liver, which is important for venous circulation. So I started taking a cup of yarrow tea every night before going to sleep, in addition to using the magnet.[7]

After two to three weeks of combining the yarrow tea and the magnet therapy, the cellulite had cleared up almost completely. From when I first started using the magnet, it took four to six weeks for my leg to be 90 percent improved.

MAGNETS AND HOMEOPATHY

Homeopathy is popular in Europe (for example, members of the British Royal Family use it), and homeopathic remedies are widely available in European pharmacies. However, homeopathy is less popular in the United States, due to a combination of factors, including the power of the American Medical Association (AMA) and a historic battle between the homeopaths and the allopaths—which the allopaths won.

Homeopathy is a very interesting way of working with illness and the body. First of all, the patient's symptoms are noted, even down to very small and apparently insignificant details, such as which side of the bed the patient likes to sleep on and whether symptoms are worse in the morning or evening. After examining this wealth of detail, the homeopath chooses a remedy, based on "provings" that have been done for the past two hundred years by thousands of dedicated homeopaths.

To make a homeopathic remedy, minute amounts of a substance are specially treated so that they become therapeutic in action. By the time the process of creating the remedy has been completed, there is no discernible trace of the original substance in the remedy. This is how homeopaths can use a substance, which in normal physical reality would be poisonous, to stimulate the body's defense when displaying similar symptoms to actual poisoning. An example is the remedy arsenicum, made from arsenic and indicated for people with digestive problems in which the symptoms are similar to those induced by arsenic poisoning. However, not all homeopathic remedies are made from poisonous substances, and many are used in similar fashion to the medicinal herbs used by a herbalist. It is thought that because the remedy operates at a more subtle level, through energy rather than matter, it is able to have a deeper and more long-lasting effect.

In creating the remedy, the initial substance is diluted many times and shaken (succussed) a certain number of times with each dilution. The liquid that remains is considered to have been potentized. The more times the remedy has been diluted and succussed, the more deep-acting it is considered to be. Different dilutions are used for different levels of illness. When taken by the patient, the remedy stimulates the body's own healing response; it kicks this natural mechanism into action. A natural healing process can then take place, with no side effects and with the possibility of a complete cure.

From a conventional scientific viewpoint, the actual mechanism by which homeopathy works is still mysterious, although recent developments in quantum physics may help explain how a substance that has been diluted out of physical existence leaves an energetic fingerprint that can stimulate healing.

Three of the remedies used by homeopaths are prepared from magnets—a north-pole remedy, called *Magnetis Polus Arcticus* (M-Arct.); a south-pole remedy, called *Magnetis Polus Australis* (M-Aust.); and a bipolar remedy, called *Magnetis Poli Ambo* (M-Ambo), meaning "whole magnet." The magnet remedies belong to a class of remedies known as the Imponderables, which include X-ray, Sunlight, Moonlight, and Electricity. The term "imponderabilia" refers to that which cannot be weighed (Latin *ponderare*, which means "to weigh"), measured, or evaluated with exactitude. These remedies are not made in the usual way, because there is no substance to be diluted and shaken. Instead, milk sugar is used to absorb the energy of the imponderable in question: The milk sugar is placed in strong sunlight or moonlight or an electrical current is applied to it. In the case of magnets, the milk sugar is placed next to a strong magnet for a predetermined amount of time. The sugar is then potentized by the usual dilution and succussion (shaking) process to distill out the energy of the remedy.

Sue Mann, a homeopath living in Germany, has written an excellent essay, entitled "Magnet Therapy," on the use of magnets in homeopathic medicine, from which much of the information on homeopathic magnet remedies in this section is extrapolated.[8] A controversial remedy, magnet was not included in the early homeopathic *Materia Medica* (the homeopathic bibles that describe remedies and the symptoms for which they are used), but later works have broken through the bias against magnet as a remedy.

It is hardly surprising that magnet should find its way into the homeopathic pharmacy. Dr. Samuel

Hahnemann (1755–1843), the founder of the homeopathic method, was strongly influenced by both
Paracelsus and Mesmer (see chapter 2). However,
Hahnemann himself did not think of potentizing magnet
(this was done later by an American homeopath named
Samuel Swan [1815–1893]); instead, Hahnemann used
actual magnets to affect the energy of the patient.

In line with some of today's opinions about polarities, Hahnemann said, "A mild disposition or a tendency to chilliness . . . directs the practitioner first to
the north pole." Hahnemann considered that, in general, the north pole represented passivity, and the south
pole represented activity. He believed that magnetic
energy was enormously powerful.[9]

> [Hahnemann] recommended that the pole, selected
> of course according to its similarity to symptoms of
> the patient, was only to be touched for a minute or
> even half a minute. If, after this first dose, some rem-
> nants of the disease still remained, then one could
> consider repeating the dose a second time. The
> effectiveness of a dose of magnet usually lasted for
> over 10 days. If one made a mistake in prescribing
> magnet and needed to [use an] antidote, then one
> could apply a small electrical double-spark from
> time to time, or one could place the palm of [his or
> her] hand on a plate of zinc for half an hour.[10]

Either we have become desensitized to the power
of magnets or Hahnemann's patients were highly sug-
gestible, because these days people seem to need rather
more than 60 seconds of exposure to experience a beneficial effect. There are cases in the homeopathic literature that sound like pure placebo, such as a man who
touched his finger to a magnet for ten minutes and went
on to make a complete recovery from chronic urinary
problems.

Today homeopaths use potentized magnets, made in the manner described above. The north pole of the magnet (M-Arct.) is used to treat premenstrual anxiety, mental slowness and excess caution, nosebleeds, toothache, face and jaw pain, headache, illusory sense of smell, trembling of the feet, and chilliness. Some of these symptoms, notably the pain and feet problems, correspond to the same symptoms for which actual magnets (rather than potentized essence of magnet) are often used. The south pole of the magnet (M-Aust.) is used for mental irritability and premenstrual restlessness, styes, ear pain, dreams of fire, and a symptom the Victorians eloquently termed the "forsaken feeling".[11] Like the north pole, the south pole is indicated in cases of pain in the face and teeth. M-Aust. is probably most well-known for its success with ingrown toenails, as there are many examples in the homeopathic literature of its success with this annoying complaint.

Whole magnet (M-Ambo.) is used for burning, shooting pains throughout the body, for "headache as if a nail were driven in," and for "tendency of old wounds to bleed afresh." It is indicated when someone talks aloud to him- or herself without being aware of it or when someone is hurried, heedless, and forgetful and acts unintentionally. It is also indicated for back pain, particularly of the sacrolumbar area on waking and from stooping during the day.[12]

Modern homeopaths have discovered that the magnet remedies are useful in the treatment of children with dyslexia. The main diagnostic hint in the old homeopathic books that led to the choice of this remedy was "mind-slowness in work". Such children often show polarities in behavior, swinging between being peaceful and contentious and between achieving high and low grades at school.[13,14]

MAGNETS AND MANIPULATION THERAPIES

Increasing numbers of chiropractors and osteopaths are recommending the use of magnets to their patients, usually as additional care between treatments. By using magnets, patients can cut down on the amount of sessions needed and speed up healing time. For people with chronic aches and pains for whom manipulation methods help keep life bearable, sleeping on a magnetic mattress pad can be a great help and may cut down on the need for frequent body work treatments.

For acute injuries, magnets can make a difference in the length of time it takes to heal. When my friend Katy broke a small bone in her foot, she called her chiropractor for advice. "Put a magnet inside the bandage," he said, "as directly on the broken bone as you can manage." She did as he suggested, sliding an 800-gauss alternating-pole magnet under the elastic bandage. The doctor she had seen in the hospital where the break was x-rayed had told her that her foot would be painful and too tender to walk on for seven days. In fact, Katy was walking after four days and was back at work three days later.

MAGNETS AND DENTAL CARE

Magnets have become popular as an adjunct pain reliever in dental care. Some practitioners have found that magnets aid in the healing of the gums and jaw after dental surgery, accelerating the healing time. These practitioners find that magnets appear to increase circulation so that intractable infections and swelling can heal without needing further complicated surgery.

Patricia's experience is a good example of this kind of dental case. For her, magnet therapy proved extremely useful and enabled her to avoid additional painful and costly dental work. A dental hygienist by profession,

Patricia experimented with a magnet when she had a difficult tooth problem of her own. She had had a tooth prepared for a crown and the dentist had had to drill very deep into the tooth. After the dental work had been done, she was in a lot of pain.

> When a tooth hurts that badly after a crown preparation, you can't have the permanent crown put on until the inflammation has cleared up. If it doesn't clear up, you have to have a root canal, which I really didn't want to do. I can't take anti-inflammatory painkillers because they give me stomach problems, so I was really stuck.

Patricia's husband, a contractor, had recently experimented with using a magnetized elbow wrap for his tendinitis, with great success. Patricia, who had also heard about other dentists using magnets for tooth pain, decided to try magnet therapy on her painful jaw. She taped a 900-gauss round magnet to her cheek over the site of the problematic tooth. In addition, she took extra calcium to help the tooth heal. It took a couple of weeks to heal fully, but now, many months later, her tooth is fine and she did not have to have a root canal.

MAGNETS AND CONVENTIONAL MEDICINE

As the evidence supporting the use of magnets begins to accumulate, medical doctors are beginning to recommend magnet therapy to patients. How is this trend likely to develop? The incorporation of acupuncture into conventional medicine may give us some clues as to how magnets may be used in the future.

Increasingly, acupuncture is complementing conventional therapies. For example, doctors now sometimes combine acupuncture and drugs to control surgery-related pain.[15] Using acupuncture lowers the need for conventional painkilling drugs, thus reducing the risk of side effects for patients who take the drugs.[16,17]

Over the next few years, we can expect to see magnets used in similar ways by mainstream doctors as an adjunct to conventional painkilling medication for postoperative pain, for dental surgery pain, and perhaps increasingly for chronic pain such as that from old injuries or arthritis. There are many more ways in which magnet therapy could be integrated into conventional practices, and we will most probably witness exciting developments in this field in the future.

14

Magnets and Veterinary Medicine
The Implications for Humans

The field of veterinary medicine has been relatively quick to recognize and utilize the beneficial properties of magnets. Magnetic products ranging from leg wraps to beds designed especially for animals—particularly horses and dogs—are available through several suppliers. Horses and dogs are two types of animals often much beloved by humans and on whom we tend to spend the most money. They therefore often tend to receive the most developed forms of veterinary care.

Among sports enthusiasts, there are two that have really taken to magnets: golfers and horse owners—golfers, because golf is a sport that has an older population than any other major sport, and horse owners, because horses are vulnerable to aches and sprains. Experience has shown that horses respond very well to magnet therapy.

One of the last interviews I did for this book was with Kimberly Henneman, a veterinarian in Salt Lake City. It was one of the last interviews because it was so hard to find a time for it. Dr. Henneman is a very busy woman, with a veterinary practice that spans eight states. It's a comment on both her skill and on the nature of veterinary practice these days that she is a holistic veterinarian, using acupuncture, homeopathy, herbs, and magnets. Her experience with horses is an interesting story by itself, but the implications for human care make it compelling.

Dr. Henneman began using magnets on horses in 1991. Her first patient was a horse with a problematic scar. She first learned about magnets at a course put on by the International Veterinary Acupuncture Society (IVAS).

> To start with, I used magnets exclusively on scar tissue. I did a lot of clinical experimentation to see how magnets worked. I used unipolar magnets with the north pole primarily facing the skin. Then I started getting braver and trying [magnets] on other problems. I found that using magnets accelerated the healing process and, in some cases, allowed healing to happen when nothing else had helped. Nowadays I use magnets on sport horses any time there's any kind of achiness, on arthritis, and on acute and chronic injuries, such as tendon and ligament injuries, muscle strains, fractures, and laminitis.

Magnets have also been used on horses to treat asthma, anxiety, nerve damage, fatigue, and decreased well-being.

Much of Dr. Henneman's focus with magnets is on designing ways to attach the magnets to the horse's body so they won't come off and will be effective enough to have a therapeutic action.

> I use magnets any place where I can get them to stick or where I can make a band that will work well. I usually use 800 to 1,500 gauss for the lower leg. For the back you need deeper penetration, so I will go as high as 20,000 gauss if necessary. I often place the magnets on acupuncture points, and that is very effective, probably because there's less electrical resistance there.

Magnet therapy is not a universal panacea. If magnets don't work, we need to get more specific about what the problem is.

I asked Dr. Henneman about her success rate, and she made a clear distinction between magnets prescribed to patients and magnets that clients order from catalogs:

When I prescribe the magnets and design the treatment, the results are pretty positive. When clients go out and buy their own magnets, the results have not been quite as consistently good. But having said that, with some products I usually see good results, for example, the Norfields hock boots (400 gauss, unipolar), toe clats (800–1,000 gauss, ceramic), and bell boots. With these products, most people report that they see a difference. [These products are all specialty products for horses that horse owners order directly from catalogs.]

If magnets are used the way they are designed to be used, and if people's expectations are appropriate, then the owners are usually very happy with the results. The effectiveness of the magnets is related to level of degeneration. I see very good results with wear-and-tear problems, as long as they are not due to a biomechanical issue like poor shoeing, a problem with the rider, poor saddle-fit, a conformation problem, old scarring, or one leg being shorter than the other. If there is an underlying problem, then the magnets act like a short-term Band-Aid. In this kind of case, then, the magnets will be very good for a day or two and then become less effective. Otherwise, for wear-and-tear conditions, magnets are very successful.

I also use magnets with dogs and cats, but it's harder to use the magnets with small animals because they tend to lick them off. In my clinic, we've made mattresses out of egg crate foam, put magnets in the crevices in the foam, and placed a cover over it all. We then put this in the cage and leave it up to the animal to choose if they want to lie on it or not. The animals seem to be attracted to the magnetic pads and almost always choose to go and lie on them. Alternatively, I wrap the magnet in a bandage. I always tell people to watch the animal very closely, and if the animal appears to be bothered after a while, I suggest they remove the magnet, because the pet is probably telling you it's had enough.

I learned a lot when I had a broken foot myself, after a horse fell on me. I put a magnet on straight away, and it made the foot hurt more. So I took it off and used arnica (a homeopathic remedy) for the bruising and swelling. I waited for five days while the initial swelling went down, but my foot was still painful. Then I put the magnet back on. Within fifteen minutes, the ache was gone.

You have to pay attention to your body and its response to the magnets, and when you work with animals you have to watch them very closely to make sure the magnet isn't irritating them.

ROGACHEFSKY'S STUDY ON OSTEOARTHRITIS IN DOGS

Dr. Richard Rogachefsky, who did the gunshot wound case study detailed in chapter 8, recently completed a study on 18 dogs with osteoarthritis. The study was presented at the June 1999 meeting of the Bioelectromagnetics Society (BEMS), where it was received with much interest.[1]

The study divided the dogs into three groups. All the dogs were given a surgical procedure in the right knee that is known to induce osteoarthritis. Six were then given no treatment, six had a magnetic mattress pad put in their cage to lie on, and six had a sham pad as a control placebo. The active pad had a magnetic field surface strength of 450 to 500 gauss.

After twelve weeks the results were evaluated, and it was very clear that the dogs with the magnetic pads fared much better and suffered from markedly less degeneration than either the sham group or the non-treatment group.

Rogachefsky concluded, "This pilot study demonstrates that static magnet fields have a remarkable protective effect on articular cartilage degeneration in this animal model of osteoarthritis."

THE IMPLICATIONS FOR HUMANS

That magnets work so well on animals is a most compelling endorsement of their efficacy. Why? The fact that magnets clearly work on horses and dogs means that magnets have a therapeutic effect beyond placebo. Horses and dogs aren't vulnerable to the placebo effect. They don't know what the medicine is; they are unaffected by the pretty packaging, the claims made in the fancy pamphlet, or what the network marketing salesperson said. Horses and dogs just want to get well.

Let's look briefly at two other healing methods that work very well with these animals.

For many years, acupuncture has been used to treat animals, in particular, horses and dogs. The International Veterinary Acupuncture Society (IVAS) has approximately 1,400 members worldwide, of whom about 800 have been certified by IVAS to practice veterinary acupuncture. Certification includes a written examination, a canine practical examination, an equine practical examination, submission of case reports, and completion of 40 hours of internship with another IVAS-certified member. As we have already seen, acupuncture is closely allied with magnetic therapy, and some acupuncturists use magnets in just the same way that they use needles. So it's not particularly surprising that if acupuncture works on animals, magnets will too.

Another system of medicine that works very well with animals is homeopathy. The Academy of Veterinary Homeopathy *(www.theavh.org)* has approximately 150 practicing members in the United States. In addition, homeopathy is widely practiced by veterinarians in Europe. Over the years, I've used homeopathy (and also, more occasionally, acupuncture) on my own animals with much success. My dog loves to take homeopathic remedies and usually detests allopathic medicine. He spits out antibiotics but will roll over on his back and open his mouth for a homeopathic remedy. It's remarkable to witness, and I'm quite sure his reaction isn't because there is a small amount of sugar in the remedy, as he never seeks out sugar otherwise.

As with magnets and acupuncture, we don't understand how homeopathy works. Yet it is very useful and powerful medicine, and it is particularly effective with children, horses, and dogs. Could this be because they don't have a belief system that interferes with the healing effect?

Reverse Placebo Effect

What we may be observing with all these systems, including magnet therapy, that work so well with animals is that there is no reverse placebo effect in operation. I'm using the term "reverse placebo effect" to describe a situation in which negative belief gets in the way of the healing process.

The *placebo effect* is the term given to a situation in which cure is effective because patients believe the medicine or system of therapy is going to make them well. Patients can have a strong belief in the doctor, so they believe what he or she tells them, or they can have confidence in the method of treatment. Usually both factors conjoin. It's also been shown that if the doctor doesn't believe in the therapy, it's less likely to work.

With the reverse placebo effect, the belief system of the patient obstructs the cure. The logical adult mind has the capacity to nullify a potential method of healing. If we don't know how something works, and we don't believe it can work, we are often capable of blocking the healing effect and finding that, surprise, surprise, the medicine doesn't work.

The human mind is a very powerful instrument in the healing process. All doctors know that if the patient's will is against the treatment, healing is less likely than if the patient is fully aligned—body, mind, and soul—with the process of cure.

PHYSICS AND BELIEF SYSTEMS

Why is it hard for us to believe that these energy-based systems, such as homeopathy, acupuncture, and magnets, actually work? The answer lies in the realm of physics.

Modern thinking in the natural sciences depends on physics. Physics is concerned with the most fundamental aspects of life, such as light, heat, matter, and energy. Physicists observe these fundamental aspects of life and then extrapolate theories to explain how the physical world works. So physics is not absolute. It changes over time, depending on what scientists understand. In terms of consensus reality, physics helps delineate our view of the natural world and of what we think is possible.

A hundred years ago, scientists thought they completely understood the physical world, and then along came Albert Einstein and his theory of relativity, closely followed by Max Planck and the birth of quantum physics. Since then, physics has been undergoing a fairly continual revolution.

Before Einstein, when what is often referred to as the Newtonian worldview had precedence, matter and energy were seen as two different phenomena. Matter was definable as solid, liquid, or gas. Energy primarily manifested itself as light and heat. Einstein explained that, actually, matter and energy existed along a continuum, which meant that heat, previously thought of as an emanation of matter or even a separate element in its own right, was now seen as molecules in motion.

Max Planck found that radiant heat energy travels in particles and that there is a certain smallest particle that cannot be divided. Planck called this smallest particle a quantum. Planck's experiments were unquestionably accurate, and so physicists had to accept his quantum theory. Soon the same sort of indivisible unit—the quanta—was found in light and in electricity. In the 1920s, physicists realized that the particle theory by itself was incomplete and that there was an accompanying wave motion involved.

How Physics Influences Our View of Medicine

Physicists are still working to determine how the natural world works. Conventional remedies, such as surgery and chemical drugs, can be satisfactorily explained by basic mechanistic physics. Other systems of medicine, such as acupuncture, homeopathy, and magnets, cannot. These systems seem to work at a level of reality that coincides more with quantum thinking than with Newtonian physics.

In homeopathy, there are no detectable molecules of the healing substance remaining in the remedy. From a Newtonian perspective, a homeopathic remedy simply consists of sugar and water. The fact that homeopaths claim that the remedy now contains the energy of the original substance is meaningless from a Newtonian perspective. In addition, the idea that the healing agent is the same as a substance that would have given you the symptoms from which you now suffer makes no sense.

Magnets are also mystifying from a Newtonian perspective. Dr. Kim Henneman said, "It looks as though magnets stimulate changes in electrolytes and changes in blood circulation—there's clearly an effect upon fluids—but how they do that appears to depend on some mechanisms that we haven't appreciated yet, maybe involving neuropeptides."

One of the more recent developments in quantum physics is string theory, which is sometimes referred to as M theory. (M theory is an amalgam of five string theories.) This amazing theory operates in a seven-dimensional reality and shows that when you get into subatomic realms, the smallest, indivisible components of the universe are not particles but infinitesimally small loops that resemble tiny vibrating strings.

Dr. Henneman commented, "[String theory] would explain why a homeopathic remedy works. Shaking the remedy is like strumming a chord. The chord has a particular resonance, which is transferred into the water. Magnets fall into this same category of energy medicine, what we might call vibrational medicine. The actual mechanism we haven't yet begun to understand." And she's right about that. We still don't fully understand how magnets affect the physiology of the body. Chapter 15 investigates all the different theories about how magnets might work, in the light of all the most recent scientific evidence.

Part 4

Theories
and Speculation

15

Possible Explanations

So far in this book, I've described the many ways magnets are being used to treat various conditions. I've also discussed much of the available scientific literature on the subject. We've seen that double-blind studies, anecdotal reports, and the experiences of a variety of physicians show that magnets do indeed have a therapeutic effect, especially to relieve pain and reduce inflammation.

The big question is, how do magnets work in order to generate this therapeutic effect? What effect do they have on the physiology of the body? The simple answer is that we don't know. No one knows exactly what magnetic fields do to the body. There are several theories, and many pieces of the puzzle are beginning to emerge, but a crystal clear understanding of how magnetic fields affect the body has yet to manifest.

This chapter describes and, to some extent, evaluates the current theories on how magnetic fields affect human physiology, how scientists are thinking about this issue at the moment, and where all this investigation might take us.

Once we agree that magnets do work, then we have all the more reason to find out how and why. This question of how magnets work has ideological as well as practical implications. It is a question that everyone working in the field would love to be able to answer. Looking for the solution to this question leads science into some fascinating territory and may help us understand the physiology of the body at a deeper, subtler level.

Understanding the mechanism by which magnetic fields interact with the cellular structure of the body could lead to cures for such problematic diseases as cancer and arthritis. Uncovering this mechanism will probably also lead to a discovery of the mechanism that governs other subtle energy forms of healing.

As I've written elsewhere in this book, medical science has been somewhat dominated by the chemical and molecular framework. The atomic or subatomic "energy" reality of the body has not been studied as deeply as chemical processes have. The same is true for methods of medical treatment that function at this level. However, this situation is changing. Quantum physics and the rise in popularity of physical remedies (such as acupuncture and magnets) are influencing medical thinking toward a physics- and atomic-based perspective. The study of magnetic fields falls under this matrix of ideas and knowledge.

There are various theories that attempt to explain how magnet therapy works. It feels a bit like living during the time before electrical current could be measured. We know there's something going on with the electromagnetism of the body, but we can't completely measure it yet. And we certainly can't see it. But we are probably quite close to understanding the truth.

Perhaps in the next few years we will see a breakthrough in our ability to measure and detect the electromagnetic field and activity of the body. Once this happens, we will be able to photograph the aura more accurately, see acupuncture points, see the energy field of a homeopathic remedy interacting with the patient's own field, and find out why these remedies work and how they can be improved by the application of modern science. Perhaps we'll be able to place a magnet on the body and watch a change occur in the electromagnetic field of the patient. We don't have such sophisticated tools yet, so we still live in the land of conjecture and theory.

This is what is known: Dr. Marko Markov wrote in 1997, "It is clear now that endogenous electromagnetic and magnetic interactions are associated with many basic physiological processes, ranging from ion-binding and molecular conformation in the cell membrane to the macroscopic mechanical properties of tissues."[1] This means that we know that the body itself (which is what *endogenous* means) generates electromagnetic and magnetic impulses to perform a wide range of functions. We also know that externally generated magnetic and electromagnetic fields have an effect on the body.

In the report of her study on magnets and fibromyalgia, Dr. Agatha Colbert stated, "There is no longer any doubt that weak electromagnetic and static magnetic fields can modulate biochemical processes in biological tissue in a physiologically meaningful manner."[2] What we don't know is exactly how this happens.

The Baylor Study report said cautiously:

> We cannot explain the significant and quick pain relief reported by our study patients. The effect could result from a local or direct change in pain receptors, but it is also possible that there was an indirect central response in pain perception at the cerebral cortical or subcortical areas, or a change in the release of enkephalins at the reticular system. If the magnetic fields have an impact on the subcortical level of the brain, it is possible that the application of one magnetic device in one painful area may more or less reduce the pain elicited in other trigger points.

This study coincides with mounting evidence that magnetic fields interact in significant ways with biological tissues. The exact mechanisms of the interaction of magnetic fields with biological tissues resulting in functional changes are unknown. This is particularly true for our understanding of the pain relief associated with the application of a magnetic field to trigger points as demonstrated in this study.[3]

CURRENT THEORIES

Before things get even more complicated, I'm going to attempt to decode some of the current theories. Please be aware that at this stage, much of this discussion exists at the level of rampant speculation. I will endeavor to make clear the distinctions among knowledge, useful imaginings, and sheer fantasy.

1. Stimulation of Blood Flow

When it comes to treating inflammation and wounds, magnets appear to work by stimulating blood flow. Many forms of physical therapy, such as applying hot and cold water, massage, and using ice, operate on this principle. Speed up the flow of blood, and healing happens faster. Debris in the tissue is carried away faster, and new blood comes in to nourish the damaged tissue.

Do magnets increase blood flow? And if so, how? At one time, it was suggested that an increase in blood flow occurred because the magnetism attracted the iron in the blood, thus stimulating the blood to circulate at an increased rate. Iron is contained within hemoglobin molecules in the blood. If the iron is attracted to the magnet, so the theory goes, this will increase blood flow to the area on which the magnet has been placed, thus stimulating the body's natural healing mechanism. This theory, interesting as it is from a medieval perspective, is flawed because iron in the blood is bound to hemo-globin and is not free to respond to a magnet. After all, hemoglobin is not a bunch of iron filings.

If magnetic fields were stimulating blood flow in the usual way, then there would always be reddening of the skin during and after treatment. But this is very rarely seen with magnets, and only when there is a condition of toxicity, such as Sabrina's experience with cel-lulite, described in chapter 13. In addition, there would be an experience of heat, which is, again, very rarely reported by magnet users.

Another big problem with the blood flow theory concerns timing. It has often been reported, and supported in such studies as the Baylor Study, that pain relief occurs within minutes following the application of a magnet. The theory that the magnet enhances the blood flow and therefore diminishes inflammation and pain, resulting in less pain, is not a sufficient explanation for the very dramatic pain relief that is often felt in too short a time to be caused by increased blood flow. The results of this study, instead, support the next theory.

2. Magnets Stimulate the Release of Endorphins

As we know from studies on acupuncture (see chapter 12), by stimulating acupuncture points, you can influence neurotransmitters to the brain and cause the release of endorphins, which create a sense of well-being and reduce sensations of pain.

This theory explains (or begins to explain) how magnets can be helpful in depression, how they generate a sense of well-being, and how they relieve pain. However, it doesn't explain how magnets reduce inflammation or speed up the healing of wounds.

Is there some mechanism that lies beneath both the nervous system and the blood circulation? Is there some realm common to both that perhaps magnets stimulate?

Is there some mechanism, which once stimulated, can improve the function of all cells in the affected area, thus stimulating blood flow and signal transduction, with all the healing capacity of the body marching to the same tune, the same resonance, the same influence?

3. The Cell Membrane Theory

Most people working in the field of biophysics agree that the most likely aspect of physiology influenced by magnetic fields is the cell membrane. The trouble is, there is a variance of opinion and conjecture about just what exactly happens at the cell membrane and what happens next.

When I asked Arthur Pilla how he thinks magnets work, he replied:

> Our first theory, way back in the early seventies, was that the cell membrane was the obvious target for pulsing magnetic fields. We thought that the reason for this was because the cell membrane contains lots of ions that are bound, either partly or tightly, to molecular sites. Enzyme kinetics showed us that ions performed a regulating function. In other words, you bind an ion to an enzyme, and it activates the enzyme. This causes something else to happen biochemically, and this sets into motion a whole cascade of events.
>
> The bioelectromagnetic community is pretty convinced at this point that the cell membrane or other internal cell surfaces that form electrified interfaces with the body fluids in which they are bathing are the target for magnetic stimuli. More than likely, it will be a particular ion or ligand that binds to a certain molecular site that then activates the molecule. What we do when we apply a magnetic field is modulate the rate of binding, and this can speed up fracture repair or reduce swelling, for example.

So we're pretty convinced that cell surfaces in general are the targets and that simple ions probably are affected.

Note that Pilla referred to "the cell membrane or other internal cell surfaces." When I asked which one it was, he said he didn't know—nobody knows. But he continued, leading to speculative mechanism number four.

4. Calcium Binding

According to Dr. Pilla:

> There's clear data on calcium binding to a molecule called calmodulin, which is a ubiquitous regulatory molecule on many cellular systems. In my lab, we have shown that a very weak static field can affect that molecule. So we know for sure that magnetism affects the rate of calcium binding. That then changes the speed at which something can happen, overall.

If magnets induce the migration of calcium ions, then this may explain how magnetic fields help bone healing. This theory suggests that magnets may also be effective at disposing of the excessive calcium deposits found in arthritis.

5. Ion Exchange at the Cell Wall

Some people have taken the cell membrane/calcium binding theories and constructed a theory based on the idea of negative ionization. I heard Dr. Ernest Vandeweghe lecture on this theory at a conference put on by the Nikken corporation. Although the science in this theory is simplistic, it does offer some explanation of why some people feel better after sleeping on a magnetic mattress pad.

Vandeweghe, a doctor of pediatrics at UCLA Medical Center, has been using magnets since 1973 and is currently on the advisory board to the Nikken corporation.

Over the years that he has been working with magnets, Dr. Vandeweghe has never seen any toxicity or negative side effects from using permanent magnets or electronic magnet therapy. On the contrary, he has seen a wide range of therapeutic benefits. From this clinical evidence, he concluded that magnets must affect the whole body and, therefore, every cell in the body. In addition, because they have no side effects, magnets must be doing something that happens naturally.

Vandeweghe concluded that magnets must function at the level of the cell, repairing the damage to cellular uptake and elimination that happens over the course of a day, building the cell back up at night. This mechanism, by which molecules pass in and out of cells, nourishing them and cleansing them, is dependent on ions at the cell wall, which allow the cell to be permeable. During the day, the number of these ions decreases. Sleep restores them, and, according to this theory, so do magnets. This may be why people feel more vital and need less sleep when they use magnetic mattress pads and wear magnetized foot insoles.

Veterinary doctor Brad Gordon gave another description of this mechanism on the Web site Medicinegarden.com:

> [The] resting electrical potential . . . is maintained and regulated by the cell membrane of each cell. This electrical potential is necessary for normal cell metabolism and function. If a cell has no electrical potential, it is nonfunctional and dead. Cell membranes control these potentials by utilizing charged particles called ions. The potential of a cell is proportional to the ion exchange and ion regulation going on at the cell membrane. This ion

exchange and ion regulation is responsible for the oxygen utilization of the cell. . . . Magnetic field therapy influences and enhances the ion exchange at the cell membrane level, thus "encouraging" a return of normal cell function and improved cell utilization of oxygen.

At Healthtechnologies.com, we find that the ion theory is again put forward:

To operate at peak efficiency, our bodies prefer a negative ion (cation) environment. But as we move about during the day, we build up positive ions (anions) as static electricity. Magnets help to restore a healthy cation concentration. Thus we can wear magnets on our bodies at places of high blood flow to feel better, elevate mood, increase energy, and boost our immune system. Also, because healing is accelerated with cations (−), placing a magnet over a painful area will usually relieve pain as well as promote healing. This is most dramatically observed in the control of carpal tunnel syndrome. Because the blood vessels in the wrist are so close to the skin and transport a high volume of our blood in a short time, bracelets are an excellent delivery system for magnetic energy generally, and specifically in the control of wrist-related problems. In short, when you want to control pain in a specific region of the body, put a magnet over it. If you want a whole-body bathing of cationic (−) charge for increased wellness, put the magnet over a very vascular region such as the wrist or neck.

There's no proof for any of this (in particular, that last idea about using a magnetic bracelet or necklace has not, so far, been borne out by studies), but it all makes for interesting speculation.

6. Magnets Influence Cell Water and Accompanying Cell Biochemistry

According to the Baylor Study:

> We are interested in the possible role of water in the pain mechanism, and attempts will be made to evaluate the physical basis of this idea using magnetic resonance technology. It is now clear that water is organized in space and time, and in a human study conducted by one of us (Carlton Hazlewood), subjective pain relief was associated with a shift of T-cells into the S-phase. Beall and colleagues demonstrated cyclical changes in the physical state(s) of water with the water being most organized in the S-phase. That water plays a major role in explaining the therapeutic effects of magnetic fields has also been proposed by others.

When I asked Dr. Hazlewood if he had a hypothesis about how permanent magnets work, he responded:

> Yes. A pain receptor site is really an electromagnetic entity, so the experience of pain may well be a major electromagnetic event in the body. Magnetic fields could be a conductor, by direct magnetic field interaction with the electromagnetic mechanistic properties of a receptor site. People say, "Oh, but the magnetism doesn't go into the body," but this isn't so. Molecules are not quiescent; they are replete with motion. The magnetic field can activate a receptor site in the same manner that the receptor molecule would. This is a hypothesis that needs to be tested.

7. Low-Amperage Current Theory

We know from Becker's work that a low-amperage current flows down the outside of the nerve sheath via the gliel calls that line the outside of the nerves. When there is injury or disease, these gliel cells transport a low-amperage current to the traumatized area to create an electrical environment whereby cell walls become more permeable. When the cell wall is more permeable, it is easier to get inflammatory material out of the cell and to get nutrients in.

In his paper on using magnetic foot insoles for the treatment of diabetic peripheral neuropathy, Dr. Weintraub wrote:

> The magnetic foot insole devices (Magsteps by Nikken) used in the study were permanent[ly] bonded polymers with a 475 gauss steep field gradient. These insoles are constructed so that both poles are active in a geometric multipolar triangular arrangement. This produces a low-level, submaximal magnetic field. This field penetrates 1.75 inches (4 cm). When blood vessels and nerves come into contact with these alternating magnetic poles, a current is induced via the movement of negative and positive ions. This is a restatement of Faraday's Law of movable excitable tissue in a static magnetic field inducing the equivalent of time variation.

Currently, other researchers in the field view Weintraub's explanation as interesting but unlikely.

8. Magnets Balance the Body's Electromagnetic Field

As I discussed in chapter 3, some people (notably Dr. Nakagawa of Japan) believe that using magnets can help compensate for insufficient access to the earth's electromagnetic field and overexposure to human-made electromagnetic fields. The theory goes that many symptoms are caused by Magnetic Field Deficiency Syndrome and that using magnets reverses this problem. There are no credible scientific data to back up this claim, but there are some anecdotal reports that suggest a relationship between electromagnetic field exposure and the use of magnets.

Early on in the research phase of this book, Jessica, an old friend, called to shoot the breeze. I told her that I was investigating magnet therapy. I should have known what she would say next: "Magnets!" she said. "They've changed my life!"

Jessica is a multimedia artist who was a computer programmer for many years. She now freelances, building state-of-the-art Web sites for major companies from her home office. She spends many hours in front of computers and various accompanying electronic machines every day. She has been working with computers for more than three decades. Over the years, she has come to realize that despite the fact that she loves her work, something in all her equipment makes her feel tired and drained. "It isn't just because I sit still for long periods of time. I do stretch and go for walks during the day. For whatever reason, my system is very sensitive to the electromagnetic waves from the computer. These electromagnetic emanations make me exhausted."

At the suggestion of a friend, Jessica decided to try wearing magnetic insoles in her shoes while she worked. She was amazed to find that they made a significant difference. "There's no doubt in my mind. When I wear the magnetic insoles, I feel more aligned and grounded, and I don't get that strange exhausted feeling. I don't get as much energy drained off of me while I am working."

Somehow, wearing magnets helps Jessica's body stay in a state that, to her, feels like wellness. If she doesn't wear the magnetic insoles, by the end of the day she feels drained. But if she does wear them, the state of wellness is maintained throughout the day. She identifies the causative factor of the unwell feeling as being the electromagnetic emanations of the computer. She doesn't get this "strange exhausted" feeling when she is out hiking in the hills all day, sitting by the fire reading a book, or even sitting in boring meetings. The strange feeling affects her globally, and when she uses the magnets she feels generally well, which suggests that the magnetic field induced by the magnetic insoles affects her whole body.

If we accept Jessica's version of reality for a moment and believe her perception of her world, we have to conclude that the magnets are doing something to her whole system and probably to the electromagnetic field of her own body. Somehow the magnets keep her own electromagnetic field aligned so that it doesn't get knocked out of balance by the electromagnetism of the computer equipment.

9. The "Magnets Are Placebo" Argument

Some people think that magnets are pure placebo, that the power of suggestion is all that is at work here. But the double-blind studies by the Baylor team, by Colbert, and by Man conclusively show that magnets can have a therapeutic result beyond that of placebo. In addition, magnets are usually not dispensed by a physician or figure of authority, which somewhat cuts down on their placebo potential. They also do not come in the form of a pill or other recognized form of medicine.

Most people don't take kindly to newfangled forms of medicine, preferring tried-and-true methods. The fact that magnets are weird and new and that you can buy them in places that don't feel at all medical, such as Kmart, may work against any placebo effect, rather than the other way around. Finally, as mentioned earlier, magnets are effective in animals, which are unaffected by the usual placebo stimuli on humans.

SUMMARY

So, that's the current range of thinking about how magnets work to relieve pain and alleviate certain symptoms. As you can see, behind these different opinions, there is the glimmering of a satisfactory understanding. Given all the attention focused on this matter right now, it's highly likely that in the near future some breakthrough will clarify the mechanism by which magnets work therapeutically on the body.

16

Conclusion
The Future of Magnets

As I said in chapter 1, when I started working on this book, I knew next to nothing about magnets. I have a background in physiology and in energy medicine from years of training and practicing acupuncture, which has helped me know what questions to ask. And I was interested in this phenomenon of magnets, with its wealth of anecdotal support. Once I started hearing so many stories from satisfied magnet users, I knew that something curious and potentially very important was taking place. My background gives me enough experience to know that current scientific consensus has some blind spots and certainly doesn't reflect everything there is to know about health and healing.

Conversely, I've witnessed enough quackery (mostly well-meaning) in the past twenty years to think that we do indeed need protection from wacky forms of medicine that are unproven either by centuries of use or by well-designed clinical trials.

During the nine months it took to research and write this book, I talked to scientists and researchers investigating magnetism and its effect on human physiology. I talked to doctors, acupuncturists, and other medical professionals using magnets on their patients; to businesspeople who manufacture and sell magnets and magnetic devices; and to people who have used magnets on themselves, with or without medical super-vision. The information in this book is largely the result of these conversations.

I asked some of these people what they thought about the future of magnet therapy. The biophysicist Arthur Pilla said:

> I'm very excited. When I first started in this work, I had many big dreams. I thought we'd be using magnetic fields in cancer research by this point, even as a therapy for treating cancer. We haven't got that far yet. For a while, everything came to a standstill. The industry that grew up around the bone-growth stimulators for the difficult-to-heal fractures was overtaken by venture capitalists and businesspeople and ceased to be innovative. The FDA played a big role in reducing innovation because of the cost of doing clinical trials and the vagaries of the FDA. It was all very frustrating to me, but now I see this field reemerging. The whole field of electromagnetic research is getting reborn. It was complacent for many years, but now, with all the interest in static magnets, it's back again, and there's funding coming in for research. That's a great boon for us scientists.

Agatha Colbert, the physician/acupuncturist and author of the study on fibromyalgia detailed in chapter 6, sounded a cautious note when she said, "There's a lot of hype about magnets at the moment. I think magnet therapy works a lot like acupuncture in the sense that it nudges along the body's own healing mechanism. It's not going to be miraculous, but it may accelerate heal-ing. Magnets definitely alter the electromagnetic field of the body and, in so doing, trigger the healing response."

With this caution in mind and without touting magnets as a miracle cure, I found that everyone I spoke with agreed that magnets do work when used correctly under the right conditions. This fact has the potential to be revolutionary in health care.

What are the ramifications of millions of people finding that magnets help to ease their pain and alleviate the symptoms of various other ailments? There are several. First, many people will find relief without having to use painkillers and anti-inflammatory drugs, thus avoiding both expense and drug side effects. Second, some people will find relief for conditions that have historically been difficult to treat, such as osteoarthritis, fibromyalgia, and diabetic peripheral neuropathy. All these conditions are highly resistant to other forms of treatment. Third, there are very promising implications for the future development of medicine and for our knowledge of the human body.

Dr. Marko Markov has said, "The potential for electromagnetic fields to restore normalcy to disturbed biological systems seems enormous. Uncovering the mechanisms responsible may be a formidable challenge but offers the promise of significantly advancing our understanding of communicative processes in the body at a physical/atomic level rather than the current chemical/molecular level."[1]

Understanding these mechanisms may also help us understand how acupuncture and other forms of medicine work. It has been problematic to design research studies showing that energy-based forms of medicine, such as acupuncture and homeopathy, have a consistent effect beyond that expected from placebo. There are many reasons for this, and I refer the interested reader to a paper by Ted Kaptchuk.[2]

Due to the complexity of these medical systems and the focus on highly individualized care, it is impossible to treat every patient the same way. Yet it is precisely this criteria—the delivery of exactly the same treatment to each subject—that is necessary to satisfy current research standards.

In the case of magnet therapy, with its more gross application and simpler diagnostic procedure, it is possible to design studies that satisfy the criteria for double-blind, randomized, placebo-controlled studies. At the moment, whatever the benefits and deficits of these criteria for judging the effectiveness of medical treatments, it is the standard to which science adheres. Medical science currently speaks in the language of "randomization, blinding, and p values."[3] There may come a time when we are able to expand this system and successfully gauge the subtler methods of medicine, but for now this is our reality.

The implications are thus: if magnetic fields can be determined to have a quantifiable and therapeutic effect on the human body, then the way is paved for an understanding of how the subtler systems—acupuncture, homeopathy, hands-on healing—work. If and when this occurs, all of medical science will take a huge step forward.

Appendix
Magnets and the Law

In the United States, the FDA wields a firm hand over alternative medical practices and products. In addition, the Federal Trade Commission (FTC) controls how companies in the United States do business. If the companies step out of line regarding FDA standards, then it is the FTC that cracks down on them.

As well as policing the traditional avenues of sale, the FTC has become involved in investigating claims made on Web sites. The Internet is a new and powerful avenue for sales of health products and for the dissemination of health-related information. As of December 1998, 22.3 million adults accessed the Web seeking health and medical information. Health and medical content is the sixth most popular topic on the Web. Of all Americans, 29 percent looked to the Internet for medical information, and more than 70 percent of those were looking for information prior to visiting a doctor's office. People suffering from serious diseases, such as cancer, are particularly vulnerable to false claims made on Web sites. In general, consumers spend millions on unproven products on the Web, some of which, according to the FTC, are deceptively marketed.

In the summer of 1999, the FTC launched Operation Cure All, designed to prevent bogus claims from appearing on the Internet. For the two previous years, the FTC had conducted an annual Health Claim Surf Day. These Surf Days identified about 800 Web sites and numerous Usenet newsgroups that contained promotions for products or services purporting to help cure, treat, or prevent six diseases: heart disease, cancer, AIDS, diabetes, arthritis, and multiple sclerosis. After each Surf Day, companies of these Web sites were sent email messages, warning them that disseminating false or unsubstantiated claims violates federal law.

After surveying a representative sample of the 1998 sites, the FTC found that 28 percent of the sites had either removed their claims or had been taken down entirely. A spokesperson for the FTC said that the agency was very encouraged by the fact that company Web masters of more than a hundred sites making questionable claims had voluntarily cleaned up their Web sites. However, some did not. So in 1999, with Operation Cure All, four sites were named as having made deceptive claims; two of these were selling magnetic products.

Magnetic Therapeutic Technologies, Inc. (MTT) claimed that their magnetic devices could help in the treatment of cancer, HIV, and other health problems. MTT agreed to a consent order, prohibiting them from making these claims and any similar unsubstantiated claims for magnetic therapy products and any other products.

Pain Stops Here! Inc. (PSH) also promoted magnetic therapy devices and made disease treatment claims for its devices. The FTC said that this company operates in a similar manner as MTT. PSH was claiming that its magnet therapy devices were effective in treating a variety of ailments, including cancer, liver disease, and arthritis. As with MTT, PSH had to sign a consent order prohibiting them from making similar unsubstantiated efficacy claims for magnetic therapy products, as well as any other product or program. The order also prohibited PSH from misrepresenting the results of any scientific studies or research.

It is important to note that out of the four worst offending Web sites, two were selling magnetic products. This suggests that the unscrupulous are drawn to the lucrative realm of magnetic therapy products.

The FTC offered consumers the following guidelines to help in evaluating any health claim. However, do consider, when reading this list, how often respectable pharmaceutical drugs are advertised in these ways. Making exaggerated claims for medical products is a sin as old as time itself. That said, if Web sites make any of the following advertising gimmicks, be wary, especially when you are thinking about whether to use a health-care product.

1. If it sounds too good to be true, it probably is.
2. The product is advertised as a quick and effective cure-all for a wide range of ailments.
3. The promoters use phrases like *scientific breakthrough, miraculous cure, exclusive product, secret ingredient,* or *ancient remedy.*
4. The text is in "medicalese"—impressive-sounding terminology to disguise a lack of good science.
5. The promoter claims the government, the medical profession, or research scientists have conspired to suppress the product.
6. The advertisement includes undocumented case histories claiming "amazing" results.
7. The product is advertised as available from only one source.[1]

You will see how many of the claims for magnets readily fall into many of these categories. But so does aspirin—an ancient remedy that treats a wide range of conditions and that is heralded as something of a miracle drug in certain situations. The difference is that a huge amount of research has been performed on aspirin.

As a result of the FTC crackdown, other magnet companies have become even more cautious. Nikken, Inc., refused to allow their distributors to engage in any kind of formal interview with me while I was doing the research for this book. Nikken has a policy of not speaking with any media for fear that their words will appear in print in the context of making health-related claims. Their literature is very careful to speak in terms of wellness rather than health. In an extraordinary feat of wordplay, the word "magnet" barely makes an appearance in the Nikken catalog, even though practically all their products contain magnets. Instead of the words "magnet" or "magnetic", they use the terms "Advanced Kenko technology" or "wellness technology".

In the United Kingdom, medical products are controlled by acts of Parliament, the most recent being the Medicines Act of 1968. This act did not specifically mention magnets, which gives magnet suppliers a loophole that allows them to make medical claims without infringing the law. However, these companies are being prevented from advertising by the Advertising Standards Authority (ASA), which regulates what can and cannot be claimed in advertising. The ASA has stated that suppliers of magnetic bracelets and necklaces must not claim that the products relieve pain, because there is no proof that this is true.[2] In June 1999, in a move similar to that of the FTC, the Institute of Trading Standards in the United Kingdom forced the removal of several Web pages that were making medical claims for magnets.

Notes

CHAPTER 2

1. In researching the history of magnets, I came across several assertions that struck me as dubious. I found that, as is so often the case, original blunders in earlier works had continued to be reported as fact in subsequent books. I have tried to avoid that pitfall in this book. When verification was lacking, I have noted that the report is anecdotal or legendary in nature.
2. *Compton's Encyclopedia*, <http://www.optonline.com/comptons/index.html>.
3. Pamphlet on magnets for practitioners, American Association of Oriental Medicine. Available from AAOM, 433 Front Street, Catasauqua, PA 18032 or <http://www.aaom.org/pubs.html>.
4. Ibid.
5. Ibid.
6. Ibid.
7. Information from personal communication with James Moran, acupuncturist.
8. Michael Tierra, *Biomagnetic and Herbal Therapy* (Twin Lakes, Wis.: Lotus Press, 1997), 50.
9. Martin Cannon, "The Pre-History of Mkultra," *MindNet Journal* 1, no. 99 (1997), <http://www.visitations.com/mindcontrol/mkultra.htm>.
10. Wilhelm Reich (1897–1957), Austrian psychoanalyst and bio-physicist. In his most famous work, *The Function of the Orgasm* (1927), Reich argued that the orgasm was an important component of mental and physical health. In 1939, Reich fled Nazi Germany and immigrated to the United States. He developed his theory of orgone energy and designed the orgone box to build and accumulate energy. The FDA declared this device fraudulent. Reich died in prison while serving a two-year sentence for contempt of court and violation of the Food and

Drug Act. His work influenced several late-twentieth century schools of body/mind connected therapies.

11. Bryn Mawr College Web site on Trance and Trauma, <http://serendip.brynmawr.edu/Mind/Trance.html> and the *Encyclopedia Britannica,* online edition.
12. Ibid.
13. R. Macklis, Magnetic Healing, Quackery and the Debate About the Health Effect of Magnetic Fields, *Annals of Medicine* 118, no. 5 (1993): 376–383.
14. C. Thatcher, *Plain Roads to Health Without the Use of Medicine* (Chicago: Jameson and Mor, 1886).
15. David W. Ramey. Magnetic and Electromagnetic Therapy. *The Scientific Review of Alternative Medicine* (Spring 1998), <http://www.hcrc.org/contrib/ramey/magnet.html>.
16. Hansen KM. Some observations with a view to possible influence of magnetism upon the human organism. *Acta Med Scand* 1938; 97: 339–364.
17. C. A. Bassett, Conversations with C. Andrew L. Bassett, M.D. Pulsed Electromagnetic Fields. A Noninvasive Therapeutic Modality for Fracture Nonunion (Interview), *Orthopedic Review* 15, no. 12 (1986): 781–795.

CHAPTER 3

1. The compass reads the local horizontal component of the earth's magnetic fields and senses magnetic north. But magnetic north is changing all the time. On a map, *true* north points to the pole, whereas *magnetic* north points to magnetic north at the time the map was published. For example, the current magnetic north from the west coast of California is in the north-northeast direction and falls near Alberta, 400 miles north of the Canadian border. That's a long, long way from the North Pole.
2. United States Geological Survey, National Geomagnetic Information Center, <http://geomag.usgs.gov/frames/geodynamo.htm>.
3. The first clinical trial of this technique is taking place at the Barnes-Jewish Hospital, to be followed by a second, larger trial. Stereotaxis, the company that developed the system, hopes that the technique will be available within a couple of years. Source: BBC News, 23 December 1998.

4. More information on this international collaborative project can be found at Iron Biomineralization in the Human Brain, <http://www.biophysics.uwa.edu.au/magnetite.html>. Collaborators: Professor H. G. Weiser (University –Hospital-Zurich); Paola Grassi (ETH-Zurich); Professor M. D. Fuller (University of Hawaii); Dr. Tim St. Pierre (University of Western Australia); Assistant Professor John Webb (Murdoch University); Wanida Chua-anusorn (Murdoch University).
5. Paola Schultheiss-Grassi, Jon P. Dobson, H. Gregor Weiser, and Niels Kuster, *Magnetic Properties of the Heart, Spleen, and Liver: Evidence for Biogenic Magnetite in Human Organs.*
6. Interview with David Levy, *New Yorker* (6 December 1999): 78–93.

CHAPTER 5

1. Vallbona C, Hazlewood CF, Jurida G. Response of pain to static magnetic fields in post-polio patients: a double blind pilot study. *Arch Phys Med Rehabil* 1997; 78: 1200–1203.
2. J. G. Travell and D. G. Simons, *Myofascial Pain and Dysfunction: The Trigger Point Manual, Vol. 1: The Upper Extremities* (Baltimore, Md.: Williams and Wilkins, 1983).
3. J. G. Travell and D. G. Simons, *Myofascial Pain and Dysfunction: The Trigger Point Manual, Vol. 2: The Lower Extremities* (Baltimore, Md.: Williams and Wilkins, 1983).
4. Hansen KM. Some observations with a view to possible influence of magnetism upon the human organism. *Acta Med Scand* 1938; 97: 339–364.
5. Miner WK, Markoll RA. A double-blind trial of the clinical effects of pulsed electromagnetic fields in osteoarthritis. *J Rheumatol* 1993; 20: 456–460.
6. Trock DH, Bollet AJ, Markoll R. The effect of pulsed electromagnetic fields in the treatment of osteoarthritis of the knee and cervical spine. Report of randomized, double blind, placebo controlled trials. *J Rheumatol* 1994; 21: 1903–1911.
7. BIOflex® Medical Magnetics, Inc., 3370 NE 5th Avenue, Oakland Park, FL 33334.
8. Vallbona C, Hazlewood DF, Jurida F. Response of pain to static magnetic fields in post-polio patients: a double blind pilot study. *Arch Phys Med Rehabil* 1997; 78: 1200–1203.
9. Ibid.
10. Baylor College of Medicine press release, 3 November 1997.

11. James D. Livingston, Magnetic Therapy: Plausible Attraction, *Skeptical Inquirer* (July/August, 1998).

CHAPTER 6

1. Wolfe F, Ross K, Anderson J, Russell I, Hebert L. The prevalence and characteristics of fibromyalgia in the general population. *Arthritis Rheum* 1995; 38: 19–27.
2. Colbert AP, Markov MS, Banerji M, Pilla AA. Magnetic mattress pad use in patients with fibromyalgia: a randomized double-blind pilot study. *Journal of Back and Musculoskeletal Rehabilitation* 1999; 13: 19–31.
3. Wolfe F, Smythe HA, Yunus MB, et al. The American College of Rheumatology 1990 criteria for classification of fibromyalgia: report of the Multicenter Criteria Committee. *Arthritis Rheum* 1990; 33: 160–172.
4. Vallbona C, Hazlewood CF, Jurida G. Response of pain to static magnetic fields in post-polio patients: a double blind pilot study. *Arch Phys Med Rehabil* 1997; 78: 1200–1203.
5. Weintraub MI. Magnetic bio-stimulation in painful diabetic peripheral neuropathy: a novel intervention—a randomized, double-placebo crossover study. *Am J Pain Manag* 1999; 9: 8–17.
6. Burckhardt CS, Clark SR, Bennett RM. The Fibromyalgia Impact Questionnaire—development and validation. *J Rheumatol* 1991; 18: 728–733.
7. Moldofsky H, Liu FA, Mously C, Roth-Schechter B, Reynolds WJ. The effect of Zolpidem in patients with fibromyalgia: a double-blind, placebo-controlled, modified crossover study. *J Rheumatol* 1996; 23: 529–533.
8. Carette S, McCain GA, Bell DA, Fam AG. Evaluation of amitriptyline in primary fibrositis: double-blind, placebo-controlled study. *Arthritis Rheum* 1986; 29: 655–659.
9. Russell IJ, Fletcher EM, Michalek JE, McBroom PC, and Hester GC. Treatment of primary fibrositis/fibromyalgia syndrome with Ibuprofen and alprazolam: a double-blind, placebo-controlled study. *Arthritis Rheum* 1989; 34: 552–560.
10. Colbert AP, Markov MS, Banerji M, Pilla AA. Magnetic mattress pad use in patients with fibromyalgia: a randomized double-blind pilot study. *Journal of Back and Musculoskeletal Rehabilitation* 1999; 13: 19–31.
11. Ibid.
12. Carette J, Bell MJ, Reynolds WJ, Haraoui B, McCain GA, Bykerk VP, et al. Comparison of amitrypline, cyclobenzaprine, and

placebo in the treatment of fibromyalgia. A randomized, double-blind clinical trial. *Arthritis Rheum* 1994; 37: 32–40.
13. Goldenberg D. Fibromyalgia syndrome a decade later. What have we learned? *Arch Intern Med* 1999; 159: 777–785.
14. Colbert AP, Markov MS, Banerji M, Pilla AA. Magnetic mattress pad use in patients with fibromyalgia: a randomized double-blind pilot study. *Journal of Back and Musculoskeletal Rehabilitation* 1999; 13: 19–31.
15. Ibid.

CHAPTER 7

1. Tectonic™ brand of magnets manufactured by Magnetherapy, Inc, Riviera Beach, Florida.
2. D. Man, The Influence of Permanent Magnetic Field Therapy on Wound Healing in Suction Lipectomy Patients: A Double-Blind Study, *Journal of Plastic and Reconstructive Surgery* (December 1999): 2261.

CHAPTER 8

1. Weintraub M. Magnetic bio-stimulation in painful diabetic peripheral neuropathy: a novel intervention—a randomized, double-placebo crossover study. *Am J Pain Manag* 1991; 9: 8–17.
2. Shaoxiang L, Zhifeng C, Jimin W, Junru W, Xiuyun Z. Magnetic disk applied on Neiguan point for prevention and treatment of cisplatin-induced nausea and vomiting. *Journal of Traditional Chinese Medicine* 1991; 11(3): 181–183. (The *Journal of Traditional Chinese Medicine* is a quarterly journal on clinical and theoretical research that is indexed/abstracted in MEDLINE. The journal is cosponsored by The China Association of Traditional Chinese Medicine and Pharmacy and The China Academy of Traditional Chinese Medicine. Distributed by the American Center of Chinese Medicine, 3121 Park Avenue, Suite J, Soquel, CA 95073 <http://www.jps. net/jtcm/profile.htm>.
3. Ibid.
4. For further details on this study, including photographs, see <http://www.supports4u.com/tectonic/studies2.htm>.
5. Lee KS. The effect of magnetic application for primary dysmenorrhea. *Kanhohak Tamgu* 1994; 3(1): 148–173.

6. Cody D, Moran J. Use of biomagnetic therapy to encourage growth in preterm neonates. *Neonatal Network* 1999; 18(6): 63–64.

CHAPTER 9

1. Don Maisch, of the EMFacts Consultancy, Tasmania, Australia, <http://www.tassie.net.au/emfacts/>.
2. Robert O. Becker and Gary Selden, *The Body Electric: Electromagnetism and the Foundation of Life* (New York: Quill/ William Morrow, 1985).
3. Bassett CA, Mitchell SN, Schink MM. Treatment of therapeutically resistant non-unions with bone grafts and pulsing electromagnetic fields. *J Bone Joint Surg* 1982; 64A: 1214–1220.
4. Miner WK, Markoll R. A double-blind trial of the clinical effects of pulsed electromagnetic fields in osteoarthritis. *J Rheumatol* 1993; 20: 456–460.
5. Trock DH, Bollet AJ, Markoll R. The effect of pulsed electromagnetic fields in the treatment of osteoarthritis of the knee and cervical spine. Report of randomized, double blind, placebo controlled trials. *J Rheumatol* 1994; 21: 1903–1911.
6. Janet Raloff, Harnessing Electric and Magnetic Fields for Healing and Health, *Science News* 156, no. 20 (1999): 316.
7. Pascual-Leone A, Rubio B, Pallardo F, Catala MD. Rapid-rate transcranial magnetic stimulation of the left dorsolateral prefrontal cortex in drug-resistant depression. *Lancet* 1996; 347: 233–237.
8. TMS for Depression: Magnetic Stimulation Contributes to Brain Research and Depression Treatment. *The Integrative Medicine Consult* 1, no. 10 (1999).
9. Tergau F, Naumann U, Paulus W, Steinhoff BJ. Low-frequency repetitive transcranial magnetic stimulation improves intractable epilepsy. *Lancet* 1999; 353: 2209.
10. Hoffman RE, Boutros NN, Hu S, Berman RM, Krystal JH, Charney DS. Transcranial magnetic stimulation and auditory hallucinations in schizophrenia. *Lancet* 2000; 355: 1073–1075.
11. Richards TL, Lappin MS, Acosta-Urquidi J, Kraft GH, Heide AC, Lawrie FW, Merrill TE, Melton GB, Cunningham CA. Double-blind study of pulsing magnetic field effects on multiple sclerosis. *J Altern Complement Med* 1997; 3(1): 21–29.
12. BBC News, 5 August 1998.

CHAPTER 10

1. Takahashi et al. The Effect of Pulsing EM Fields on DNA Synthesis in Mammalian Cell Cultures. *Experientia* 42: 185, 1986. Cited in John Upledger, *Magnets in Healthcare: A Cause for Pause* (UI Enterprises, 1999).
2. John E. Moulder, Medical College of Wisconsin, "Static Electric and Magnetic Fields and Human Health: Questions and Answers," <http://www.mcw.edu/gcrc/cop/static-fields-cancer-FAQ/QandA.html#1>.
3. Ibid.
4. United Nations Environment Programme. MF: The International Labour Organization, World Health Organization, 1987.
5. Vallbona C, Hazlewood DF, Jurida F. Response of pain to static magnetic fields in post-polio patients: a double blind pilot study. *Arch Phys Med Rehabil* 1997; 78: 1200–1203.
6. John Upledger, *Magnets in Healthcare: A Cause for Pause* (UI Enterprises, 1999).
7. National Radiation Protection Board. *Restrictions on Human Exposure to Static and Time Varying Electromagnetic Fields and Radiation.* Document of the NRPB 4, no. 5: 1–69, 1993. Cited in Moulder, <http://www.mcw.edu/gcrc/cop/static-fields-cancer-FAQ/QandA.html#1>.
8. Ibid.
9. John E. Moulder, Medical College of Wisconsin, "Static Electric and Magnetic Fields and Human Health: Questions and Answers," <http://www.mcw.edu/gcrc/cop/static-fields-cancer-FAQ/QandA.html#1>.

CHAPTER 11

1. OMS Medical Supplies, Inc., 1950 Washington Street, Braintree, MA 02184, 1-800-323-1839, <http://www.omsmedical.com>.
2. Nikken, Inc., 1-888-2-NIKKEN, http://www.nikken.com.
3. Hong CZ, Lin JC, Bender LF, Schaeffer JN, Meltzer RJ, Causin P. Magnetic necklace: its therapeutic effectiveness on neck and shoulder pain. *Arch Phys Med Rehabil* 1982; 63: 462–466.
4. Johnson K, Sanders JJ, Gellin R, Palesch Y. The effectiveness of a magnetized water oral irrigator (HydroFloss®) on plaque, calculus and gingival health. *J Clinical Periodontol* 1998; 25: 316–321.

5. The Cutting Edge Catalog™, P.O. Box 5034, Southampton, NY 11969, 1-800-497-9516, <http://www.cutcat.com>.
6. Yushio Manaka, *Chasing the Dragon's Tail* (Brookline, Mass.: Paradigm, 1995), xxxiv.
7. Collacott EA, Zimmerman JT, White DW, Rindone JP. Bipolar permanent magnets for the treatment of chronic low back pain. *JAMA* 2000; 283(10): 1322–1325.

CHAPTER 12

1. World Health Organization, *Viewpoint on Acupuncture* (Geneva, Switzerland: World Health Organization, 1979).
2. C. D. Lytle, *An Overview of Acupuncture* (Washington, D.C.: United States Department of Health and Human Services, Health Sciences Branch, Division of Life Sciences, Office of Science and Technology, Center for Devices and Radiological Health, Food and Drug Administration, 1993).
3. P. D. Culliton, "Current Utilization of Acupuncture by United States Patients" (presented at National Institutes of Health Consensus Development Conference on Acupuncture, Program and Abstracts, Bethesda, Md., 3–5 November 1997).
4. D. Brown, "Three Generations of Alternative Medicine: Behavioral Medicine, Integrated Medicine, and Energy Medicine," in *Boston University School of Medicine Alumni Report* (Fall 1996).
5. K. Senior, Acupuncture: Can It Take the Pain Away? *Molecular Medicine Today* 2, no. 4 (1996): 150–153.
6. National Institutes of Health, *Frequently Asked Questions About Acupuncture* (Bethesda, Md.: National Institutes of Health, 1997).
7. NIH Web site on acupuncture, <http://nccam.nih.gov/nccam/what-is-cam/acupuncture/acupuncture.htm>.
8. Dale RA. Demythologizing acupuncture. Part 1. The scientific mechanisms and the clinical uses. *Alternative and Complementary Therapies Journal* 1997; 3(2): 125–131.
9. C. Takeshige, "Mechanism of Acupuncture Analgesia Based on Animal Experiments," in *Scientific Bases of Acupuncture* (Berlin, Germany: Springer-Verlag, 1989).
10. J. S. Han, "Acupuncture Activates Endogenous Systems of Analgesia" (presented at National Institutes of Health Consensus Conference on Acupuncture, Program and Abstracts, Bethesda, Md., 3–5 November 1997).

11. J. Longhurst (UCI College of Medicine) and P. Li (Shanghai Medical University), UCI press release, 21 August 1999.
12. B. Wu, R. X. Zhou, and M. S. Zhou, Effect of Acupuncture on Interleukin-2 Level and NK Cell Immunoactivity of Peripheral Blood of Malignant Tumor Patients, *Chung Kuo Chung Hsi I Chieh Ho Tsa Chich* 14, no. 9 (1994): 537–539.
13. B. Wu, Effect of Acupuncture on the Regulation of Cell-Mediated Immunity in Patients with Malignant Tumors, *Chen Tzu Yen Chiu* 20, no. 3 (1995): 67–71.
14. Neil Sherman, "Picturing Acupuncture" (study by Huey-Jen Lee, M.D., chief of neuroradiology, University of New Jersey, presented at the Annual Meeting of the Radiological Society of North America, November/December 1999), <http://www.healthscout.com>.
15. National Institutes of Health Consensus Panel, "Acupuncture" (National Institutes of Health Consensus Development Statement, Bethesda, Md., 3–5 November 1997).
16. Bullock ML, Pheley AM, Kiresuk TJ, Lenz SK, Culliton PD. Characteristics and complaints of patients seeking therapy at a hospital-based alternative medicine clinic. *J Altern Complement Med* 1997; 3(1): 31–37.
17. Diehl DL, Kaplan G, Coulter I, Glik D, Hurwitz EL. Use of acupuncture by American physicians. *J Altern Complement Med* 1997; 3(2): 119–126.
18. Much of the information in this section was taken from the NIH Web page on acupuncture, <http://nccam.nih.gov/nccam/what-is-cam/acupuncture/acupuncture.htm>.
19. Stephen Birch, Introduction to *Chasing the Dragon's Tail,* by Yushio Manaka (Brookline, Mass.: Paradigm, 1995), xxiii.
20. Ibid, p. 65.
21. Ibid, p. 121.
22. Ibid, p. 77.
23. Robert O. Becker and Gary Selden, *The Body Electric: Electromagnetism and the Foundation of Life* (New York: Quill/William Morrow, 1985) 236.

CHAPTER 13

1. Michael Tierra. *Biomagnetic and Herbal Therapy.* (Twin Lakes, Wis.: Lotus Press, 1997).
2. Ibid.

3. Ibid.
4. Ibid.
5. Ibid.
6. It is unusual for a magnet to cause redness, heat, and puffiness, and in this case was probably due to toxins being eliminated.
7. Yarrow often causes allergic reactions, so it may not be the best herb to use for improving the liver's function in circulating chi. You could try milk thistle instead or other herbs that a qualified herbalist can advise you about.
8. Sue Mann, "Magnet Therapy," in full at <http://www.medicinegarden.com/Homeopathy/Magnet_Art_By_Sue_Mann.html>.
9. Samuel Hahnemann, *Organon of the Medical Art* (O'Reilly/Decker, Birdcage Books, 1996).
10. Sue Mann, "Magnet Therapy," in full at <http://www.medicinegarden.com/Homeopathy/Magnet_Art_By_Sue_Mann.html>.
11. James Tyler Kent, *Repertory of the Homeopathic Materia Medica* (Jain Publishers).
12. Vermeulen, *Concordant Materia Medica.*
13. Wim Roukema, Irresolution, Followed by Prompt Execution, *Homeopathic Links* 10 (Winter 1997).
14. Shandor Weiss, Dyslexia: A Case of Reversed Polarity, *Simillimum* 7, no. 2 (1994).
15. Lao L, Bergman S, Langenberg P, Wong R, Berman B. Efficacy of Chinese acupuncture on postoperative oral surgery pain. *Oral Surgery, Oral Medicine, Oral Pathology* 1995; 79(4): 423–428.
16. Lewith GT, Vincent C. On the evaluation of the clinical effects of acupuncture: a problem reassessed and a framework for future research. *J Altern Complement Med* 1996; 2(1): 79–90.
17. Tsibuliak VN, Alisov AP, Shatrova VP. Acupuncture analgesia and analgesic transcutaneous electroneurostimulation in the early postoperative period. *Anesthesiology and Reanimatology* 1995; 2: 93–98.

CHAPTER 14

1. R. A. M. Rogachefsky and M. S. Markov, "Treatment of Canine Osteoarthritis with a Permanent Magnetic Mattress" (paper presented at Bioelectromagnetics Society conference June 1999).

CHAPTER 15

1. Marko Markov, "Clinical Application of Magnetic and Electromagnetic Fields" (paper presented at the Ninth International Congress on Stress, Montreux, Switzerland, 16–22 February 1997).
2. Colbert AP, Markov MS, Banerji M, Pilla AA. Magnetic mattress pad use in patients with fibromyalgia: a randomized double-blind pilot study. *Journal of Back and Musculoskeletal Rehabilitation* 1999; 13: 19–31.
3. Valbona C, Hazlewood CF, Jurida G. Response of pain to static magnetic fields in post-polio patients: a double-blind pilot study. *Arch Phys Med Rehabil* 1997; 78: 1200–1203.

CONCLUSION

1. Marko Markov, "Clinical Application of Magnetic and Electromagnetic Fields" (paper presented at the Ninth International Congress on Stress, Montreux, Switzerland, 16–22 February 1997).
2. Ted Kaptchuk, "Some Thoughts on Efficacy Beyond the Placebo Effect," <http://www.acupuncture.com/Research/Kaptchuk.htm>.
3. Ibid.

APPENDIX

1. FTC Web page, <http://www.ftc.gov/opa/1999/9906opcureall.htm>.
2. BBC News, 9 June 1999.

Glossary

Abstract: a brief synopsis of a research study.

Acute pain: pain of recent duration that will probably completely resolve given the appropriate treatment or sometimes with no treatment at all.

Alternating current (AC): an electrical current that reverses its direction at regular, very short, intervals.

Bioelectromagnetics: a new scientific discipline that studies how living organisms interact with electromagnetic fields.

Biogenic magnetite: naturally occurring magnetite found in human organs, including the brain, heart, liver, and spleen.

Biophysics: the study of the physics of biological processes.

Case study: the detailed study of a single medical case to extrapolate possible uses for treatment methods and as a prerequisite to designing larger medical trials.

Chi (or Qi): a fundamental concept in Chinese medicine. Although it is not readily translatable into English, it can be loosely translated as the energy that flows throughout the body. Chi has several vital functions in the maintenance of health.

Chronic pain: pain of long duration that may never be entirely resolved. The goal of treatment is to successfully minimize and manage the pain and, where possible, to heal the affected area completely.

Convection: the transference of heat or mass from place to place by the circulation of fluid and the influence of gravity. Molecules move from cool regions to warmer regions of lower density.

Direct current (DC): an electric current of constant magnitude that flows in one direction only.

Double-blind: method employed in modern scientific research studies in which both researchers and subjects are kept unaware (blind) of which subjects receive real treatment and which receive placebo, or inert, treatment.

Endogenous: occurring naturally within the body.

Fibromyalgia: a disease that affects the whole body, causing widespread aches and pains, insomnia, and fatigue.

Gauss (G or g): unit of magnetic strength. 1 gauss equals 10,000 tesla. Named for Karl Friedrich Gauss (1777–1855), the German mathematician and astronomer.

Gaussmeter: instrument that measures the intensity of a magnetic field.

Hertz (Hz or hz): unit of frequency. Measures cycles per second. 1 hertz has a periodic interval (fluctuation) of 1 second. Named for the German physicist Heinrich Hertz (1857–1894), who was the first to produce electromagnetic waves artificially.

Homeopathy: system of medicine founded by Dr. Samuel Hahnemann (1755–1843) in which minute amounts of substances are used to provoke the body's own healing mechanism.

Homeostasis: the body's own tendency toward self-healing and balance.

Lodestones: naturally occurring magnetic rocks formed as a by-product of volcanic activity.

Magnetic resonance imaging (MRI): method of imaging inside the body (or the earth) developed in the 1970s. Molecules are spun by the influence of a strong magnetic field. The return of these molecules to normalcy is used to generate an image of the interior of the body.

Magnetite: a black magnetizable mineral consisting of ferrous and ferric oxides in cubic crystalline form (also called an iron spinel) ($FeO.Fe_2O_3$).

Meridians: term in Chinese medicine for the pathways in the body along which chi flows.

Oxidized: process by which another element is combined with oxygen. An oxide is a compound of oxygen with another element.

Palpating: method of medical diagnosis in which the fingers are used to feel a body part to take the pulse or read the Chinese pulses.

PEMF: pulsing electromagnetic field.

Permanent magnet: the type of magnet used in magnet therapy in which there is no electrical component. The magnetic strength is nonvarying, hence *permanent.* See also *static magnet.*

Placebo: a medical treatment that appears to be a real treatment but is actually inert, such as a pill made of starch containing no pharmaceutical ingredients.

Placebo-controlled: a research study in which there is a control group of subjects receiving treatment that looks identical to the treatment given to the study group, but that is in fact merely a placebo.

Placebo effect: the beneficial therapeutic effect that occurs regardless of the actual efficacy of the treatment. It occurs when the patient's belief and desire to recover influence the outcome of medical treatment. To offset this known phenomenon when performing a scientific research study, there must be a control group that unknowingly receives a fake version of the therapy on trial. The real treatment must achieve positive results beyond the placebo effect shown by the control group.

Potentized: when a homeopathic remedy is prepared, the active ingredient in the remedy is diluted and succussed (shaken) in order to create the required potency. Remedies are potentized to a specific numeric amount.

Pulses: Chinese method of diagnosis in which several different pulses are identified on each wrist and are considered to relate to different organs and functional systems in the body. The pulses are palpated to diagnose the specific nature of the illness, prescribe correct treatment, and then monitor the success of the treatment.

Quantum theory: theory of physics originated by Max Planck in the early twentieth century.

Randomized: a criterion of a scientific study. The selection of people taking part in the study is random.

Repeatable: a criterion of a scientific study. Scientific experiments must be able to be repeated by other scientists working with other subjects but using the identical research design to achieve a closely similar result.

Static magnets: the type of magnet used in magnet therapy in which there is no electrical component. The magnetic strength is nonvarying. See also *permanent magnet.*

Succussed: the method by which homeopathic remedies are prepared by shaking.

Tai chi: ancient Chinese exercise system that encourages the flow of chi and is said to facilitate good health and longevity.

Tesla: unit of magnetic flux density. 1 tesla equals 10,000 gauss. Named for Nikola Tesla (1857–1943), Croatian-born U.S. electrical engineer and inventor.

Theory of similars: an element of homeopathic theory stating that a miniscule amount of a substance can trigger a healing response in a patient.

Varves: sedimentary layers in the earth that can be analyzed to determine geological activity over time. Usually occurring in glacial lakes.

Bibliography

Becker, Robert O., and Selden, Gary. 1985. *The Body Electric: Electromagnetism and the Foundation of Life*. New York: Quill/William Morrow.

Becker, Robert O. 1990. *Cross Currents: The Perils of Electropollution, the Promise of Electromedicine*. New York: Tarcher/Putnam.

Bersani, Ferdinand, ed. 1999. *Electricity and Magnetism in Biology and Medicine*. New York: Klewer Academic/Plenum.

Lawrence, Ron, with Rosch, Paul, and Plowden, Judith. 1998. *Magnet Therapy: The Pain Cure Alternative*. Rocklin, CA: PrimaHealth.

Manaka, Yushio, with Itaya, Kazuko, and Birch, Stephen. 1995. *Chasing the Dragon's Tail*. Brookline, MA: Paradigm.

Matsumoto, Kiiko, and Birch, Stephen. 1986. *Extraordinary Vessels*. Brookline, MA: Paradigm.

Null, Gary, with Koestler, Vickie Riba. 1998. *Healing with Magnets*. New York: Carroll and Graf.

Payne, Buryl. 1998. *Getting Started with Magnetic Healing*. Santa Cruz: Psychophysics Press.

Tierra, Michael. 1997. *Biomagnetic and Herbal Therapy*. Twin Lakes, WI: Lotus Press.

Washnis, George J., and Hricak, Richard Z. 1993. *Discovery of Magnetic Health*. Rockville, MD: Nova.

Whitaker, Julian, and Adderly, Brenda. 1998. *The Pain Relief Breakthrough*. Boston: Little, Brown, and Company.

Index

Nikken corporation, 25
  alternating magnetic pole
    products, 152
  back-flex magnet, 135–136
  Dr. Vandeweghe and, 25,
    205–206
  foot insoles, 99, 207
  mattress pads, 139, 140
  policies, 219
  research done by, 55–56,
    58, 149
Nonunion bone fractures, 109
  Biosteogen device for, 57
  electromagnetic field ther-
    apy for, 24–25, 107,
    109–110

O

OMS (Oriental Medical
    Supply) catalog, 135,
    137, 139, 141, 147
Operation Cure All, 217–218
Orthopedic surgeons, 25
Osteoarthritis
  pulsing electromagnetic
    field (PEMF) therapy
    for, 110–111
  study on dogs, 190–191
Osteoporosis, 111

P

Pacemakers, 127
Pain relief, Baylor Magnet
    Study on. *See* Baylor
    Magnet Study
Paracelsus, 18–20
Parkinson's disease, 42, 118
Pascual-Leone, Dr., 112
Peripheral neuropathy,
    97–99
  anecdotal accounts, 11–12
  research study on magnets
    for, 97–100

Philpott, Dr. William, 62,
    147, 148, 171
Physics and belief systems,
    193–195
Pilla, Dr. Arthur, 24, 57, 78,
    96, 109, 118, 128, 146,
    148, 149, 204–205, 214
Placebo-controlled studies, 61
Placebo effect, 23, 54, 59,
    192–193
  "magnets are placebo"
    argument, 211
  reverse placebo effect,
    192–193
  veterinary medicine and,
    191–193
Planck, Max, 194
Plastic surgery. *See* Man
    study on wound healing
Plosker, Dr. Harvey, 90
Polarities, 40–41, 146–152,
    171, 173
Post-polio syndrome, 67, 68,
    128
Power spots, 35–36
Pregnancy, 126–127
Premature babies, 104–106
Products, magnetic
  bracelets and necklaces,
    140–141
  foot insoles, 5, 9, 99–100,
    138–139, 178–179,
    209–211
  jewelry, 140–141
  for magnetizing water,
    141–143
  mattress pads, 8–9, 80–82,
    139–140
  from multilevel marketing
    companies, 132–134
  polarities, 40–41, 146–152
  proper use of, 144–146

About the Author

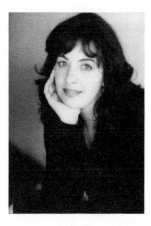

Lara Owen was raised and educated in England. After graduating from university, she spent ten years studying and practicing acupuncture and herbalism. She is a graduate of The College of Oriental Medicine, U.K., the College of Traditional Chinese Medicine in London, and the Academy of Traditional Chinese Medicine in Beijing. She cofounded one of the first multidisciplinary alternative medical clinics in Britain and was in private practice there for many years.

She then embarked on an intensive study of body-oriented psychotherapy and shamanic methods of healing, with an emphasis on women's issues. She is the author of *Her Blood Is Gold* (HarperCollins 1993), a pioneering book about the relationship between menstrual beliefs and practices and women's physical, psychological, and spiritual well-being. The book was reissued in an expanded and revised form as *Honoring Menstruation: A Time of Self-Renewal* (Crossing Press 1998).

She has lectured and taught classes internationally on several topics, including acupuncture, menstruation, and women's spirituality and creativity. She has worked in documentary film and television and appeared on radio and television in the United States and the United Kingdom. She currently lives in northern California, where she writes, teaches, and consults on a variety of projects.